NURSING MEDICAL TERMINOLOGY CHEAT SHEET

The Big Book of Nursing Medical Terminology Workbook

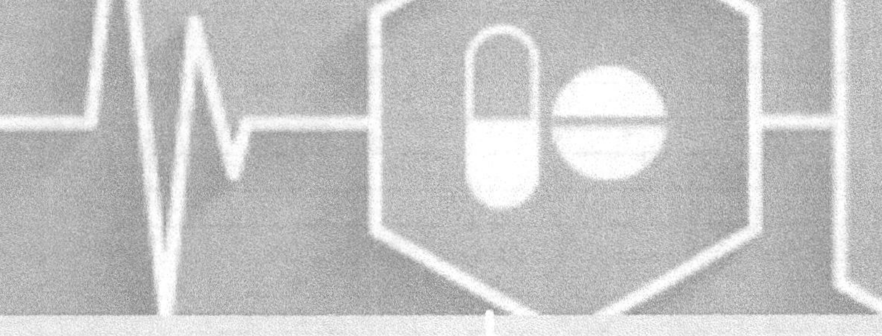

1900+ Terms	Word Search	Quiz
Test	Matching	Crosswords
Root Words	Suffixes	Prefixes

Medical Terminology 1

	Answer
diabetes mellitus	metabolic syndrome caused by insulin deficiency
diabet	r -diabetes
ic	s-pertaining to
hypotension	low bp
hypo	p- below
tens	r- pressure
ive	s- pertaining to, quality of
ion	s- condition, action
hypotensive	suffering from low bp (hypotension)
ketoacidosis	excessive production of ketones, making the blood acidic
sis	s- abnormal condition
ket/o	r/cf - ketone
acid/o	r/cf - acid
neuropathy	any disorder affecting the nervous system
pathy	s- disease
neur/o	r/cf- nerve
pneumonia	inflammation of lung parenchyma tissue
pneumon	r- air, lung
ia	s- condition
retinopathy	any disease of the retina
pathy	s- disease
retin/o	r/cf- retina of eye
tachycardia	rapid heart rate, above 100 bpm
tachy	p- rapid
card	r- heart
tachypnea	rapid breathing
pnea	r- breathe
pulmonary	pertaining to the lungs
pulmonology	study of the lungs
pulmonologist	specialist studies the lungs
ary	s- pertaining to
pulmon	r- lung
logy	s-study of
pulmon/o	r/cf - lung
logist	s- one who studies, specialist
pneumon	r- lung, air
itis	s- inflammation
respiration	process of breathing, exchange of oxygen and carbon dioxide
respir	r - to breathe
ation	s- process
atory	s- pertaining to
respiratory	pertaining to respiration (breathing)
gastric	pertaining to the stomach
gastr	r- stomach

epi	p- above
hypo	p- below
epigastric	abdominal region above the stomach
hypogastric	abdominal region below the stomach
lateral	pertaining to one side of the body
later	r- side
al	s- pertaining to
bi	p- two
uni	p- one
bilateral	pertaining to both sides of the body
unilateral	pertaining to one side of the body
macrocyte	large red blood cell
macro	p- large
cyte	r- cell
macrocytic	pertaining to the macrocyte (large red blood cell)
mature	fully developed
post mature	infant born after 42 wks gestation
premature	before expected time, eg infant born before 37 wks gestation
mature	r- fully developed
pre	p- before
post	p- after
microcyte	small red blood cell
micro	p- small
natal	pertaining to birth
nat	r- birth, born
peri	p- around
perinatal	around the time of birth
postnatal	after the time of birth
prenatal	before the time of birth
pneumothorax	air in the pleural cavity
thorax	r- chest
pneumo	r/cf - air, lung
AMI	acute myocardial infarction - heart attack
CXR	chest x-ray
ECG/EKG	electrocardiogram
IV	intravenous
cardiology	med spec of disease of the heart
cardi/o	r/cf - heart
axilla	armpit
axill	r- armpit
ary	s- pertaining to
dementia	loss of intellectual and metal functions -chronic, progressive, irreversible
de	p- without
ment	r- mind
ganglion	fluid filled cyst, or collection of nerve cells outside the brain and spinal cord
ganglion	(Greek) a swelling or knot
ileum	3rd portion of the small intestine (Latin) to twist or roll up
ilium	large wing-shaped bone at the upper and posterior part of the pelvis (Latin) groin
mucus	sticky secretion of cells in mucous membranes (Greek) slime

mucous	pertaining to mucus or the mucosa
mucosa	lining of a tubular structure that secretes
prostate	organ surrounding the urethra at base of male urinary bladder; (Greek) one who stands before
prostrate prostration (noun)	to lay flat or be overcome by physical weakness and exhaustion; (latin) to stretch out
reflex	involuntary response to a stimulus; (latin) bend back
reflux	backward flow; (latin)backward flow
septum septa (pl)	thin wall separting 2 cavities or 2 tissue masses; (latin) a partition
cervical	pertaining to the cevix, or to the neck region
cervic	r- neck
cervix	lower part of the uterus
hypertension	high BP
tens	r- pressure
hyper	p- above, beyond, excess, excessive
infusion	introduction of a substance other than blood by IV
transfusion	transfer of blood or blood component from a donor to recipient
fusion	r - to join; combining or blending of distinct bodies into one
in	p - in
trans	p - across, through
intravenous	inside a vein
intra	p- within, inside
ven	r- vein
ous	s- pertaining to
neurology	med spec of disorders of nervous system
protocol	detailed plan; as for a regimen of therapy; (latin) contents page of a book
ureter	tube that connects kidney to urinary bladder, (Greek) urinary canal, passage of urine
ur/o	urine
urethra	canal leading from bladder to the outside
uterus	organ in which an egg develops into fetus; (latin) womb
vertebra vertebrae (pl)	one of bones of spinal column; (latin) bone in the spine
abdomen	part of trunk between thorax and pelvis
abdomin	r- abdomen
anatomy	study of structures of the body
ana	r- apart from
tomy	s- process of separating
ical	s - pertaining to
anterior	front surface of the body;
anter	r - before
ior	s- pertaining to
caudal	pert to nearer the tailbone; (same as inferior, opposite of cephalic)
caud	r - tail
al	s- pertaining to
cephalic	pertaining to or nearer the head
cephal	r - head
coronal	vertical plane dividing body into anterior and posterior portions
coron	r - crown
al	s- pertaining to
distal	situated away from the center of the body;farthest from the point of attachment, refers only to limbs

dist	r - away from the center
dorsal	pertaining to the back or situated behind
dors	r - back
lateral	situated at the side of a structure
later	r- side
medial	nearer to the middle of the body
medi	r- middle
posterior	pertaining to the back surface of the body, situated behind
poster	r - back part
ior	s- pertaining to
prone	lying face down, flat on belly; (latin) bending forward
proximal	situated nearest the center of the body;situated closest to the point of attachment to the body, refers to limbs
proxim	r- nearest to the center
sagittal	vertical plane through the body divides it into right and left planes
sagitt	r- arrow
supine	lyint face up, flat on spine
transverse	horizontal plane div body into uper and lower portions (superior and inferior)
ventral	pertaining to the belly or situated nearer the face of the belly
ventr	r- belly
al	s- pertaining to
abdomin/o	r/cf - abdomen
pelv	r - pelvis
cavity	hollow space or body compartment
cav	r - hollow space
ity	s- state, condition
cranial	pertaining to the cranium (skull)
crani	r- skull
cranium	skull
diaphragm	muscular sheet separting the abdominal and thoracic cavities
diaphragm/a	r - diaphragm
quadrant	1 of 4 regions of the surface of the abdomen; 1/4 of a circle,(latin) one quarter
spine	the vertebral column, or a short bony projection
spin	r - spine
thoracic	pertaining to the chest (thorax)
thorac	r - chest
thorax	the part of the trunk between the abdomen and neck
umbilical	pertaining to the umbilicus (belly button, or the center of the abdomen
umbilic	r - navel (belly button)
umbilicus	pit in the abdomen where the umbilical cord entered the fetus
cell	smallest unit of the body capable of independent existence; (latin) storeroom
conception	fertilization of egg by sperm to form a zygote
cytology	study of the cell
cytologist	spec in the structure, chemisty, and pathology of the cell
cyt/o	r/cf - cell
fertilization	union of male sperm and female egg
fetiliz	r - to make fruitful

organ	structure with specific functions in the body
organelle	part of a cell having specialized function
organ	r - organ; (latin) intrument, tool
elle	s - small
ism	s- condition,process
tissue	collection of similar cells; (latin)- to weave
zygote	cell resulting from union of sperm and egg; (Greek) yolk
DNA	deoxyribonucleic acid- source of hereditary characteristics found in chromosomes
RNA	ribonucleic acid - the information carrier from DNA in the nucleus to an organelle to produce protein molecules
ribo	p- from ribose, a sugar
nucle	r- nucleus
steroid	large family of chemical substances found in many drugs, hormones, and body components
ster	r- solid
oid	s - resembling
anabolism	buildup of complex substances in the cell from simpler ones as a part of metabolism
anabol	r - build up
ism	s- process, condition
catabolism	breakdown of complex substances into simpler ones as a part of metabolism
chromosome	body in the nucleus that contains DNA and genes
chrom/o	r/cf - color
some	s - body
cytoplasm	clear, gelatinous substance that forms the substance of a cell, except for the nucleus
cyt/o	r/cf - cell
electrolyte	substance that, when dissolved in a suitable medium, forms electrically charged particles
electr/o	r/cf - electricity
lyte	s - soluble
hormone	chemical formed in one tissue or organ and carried by the blood to stimulate or inhibit a function of another tissue or organ; (Greek) set in motion
hormon	r- hormone
intracellular	within the cell
cellul	r - small cell
intra	p- within
lipid	general term for all types of fatty compounds; eg. cholesterol, triglycerides, fatty acids; (Greek) fat
membrane	thin layer of tissue covering a structure or cavity; (latin) parchment
membran	r - cover, skin
ous	s- pertaining to
metabolism	the constantly changing physical and chemical rocesses occurring in the cell that are the sum of anabolism and catabolism
metabol	r - change
ism	s - process, condition
mitochondria	organelles that generate, store, and release energy for cell activities
mit/o	r/cf -thread
chondr	r - granule, cartilage
-ia	s - conditionn
nucleolus	small mass within the nucleus

nucle/o	r/cf - nucleus
-lus	s - small
nucleus	functional center of a cell or structure; (latin) command center
nucle	r - nucleus
-ar	s- pertaining to
protein	class of food substances based on amino acids
arthroscopy	visual examination of interior of a joint
scopy	s - to examine, to view
arthr/o	r/cf - joint
connective tissue	supporting tissue of the body
connect	r - join together
cruciate	shaped like a cross;
ACL	anterior cruciate ligament - at front of knee,
ligament	band of fibrous tissue connecting 2 structures; (latin) band
meniscus	disc of cartilage between the bones of the joint (eg. at knee cap); (latin) cresent
muscle	tissue consisting of contractile cells
patella patellae (pl)t	thin, circular bone embedded in the patellar tendon in front of the knee joint; kneecap; (latin) small plate
patell	r - patella
therapy	systematic treatment of disease, dysfunction, or disorder
therap	r- treatment
therapeut	r- treatment
4 primary tissue groups	connective, epithelial, muscle, nervous
connective tissue	funct - bind, support, protect, fill spaces, store fat; found throughout body (eg. blood, bone cartilage, and fat
epithelial tissue	funct: protect, secrete, absorb, excrete; location- covers body surface, covers and lines internal organs, composes glands
nervous tissue	function: transmit impulses for coordination, sensory reception, motor actions; location- brain, spinal cord, nerves
histology	study of structure and function of cells, tissues, and organs
hist/o	r/cf - tissue
capsule	fibrous tissue layer surrounding a joint or other structure; (latin) little box
capsul	r - box
cartilage	nonvascular, firm connective tissue found mostly in joints; (latin) gristle
collagen	major protein of connective tissue, cartilage, and bone
coll/a	r/cf - glue
gen	s - produce, form
matrix	substance that surrounds and protects cells, is maufactured by the cells, and holds them together; (latin) mater-mother
nutrient	substance in food required for normal physiologic function
nutri	r - nourish
ent	s - end result
periosteum	fibrous membrane covering a bone
oste	r - bone
peri	p- around
um	s- tissue
synovial membrane	membrane that lines the interior of freely moving joints
tendon	fibrous band that connects muscle to bone
synovial fluid	slippery lubricant stored in the joint cavity; makes joint movement almost friction free

cardiovascular	pertaining to the heart and blood vessels
cardi/o	heart
vascul	blood vessell -r
digestion	breakdown of food into elements suitable for cell metabolism
digest	break down food -r
ive	pertaining to - s
endocrine	a gland that produces an internal or hormonal substance
endo	within - p
crine	to secrete -r
homeostasis	maintaining the stability of a system or the body's internal environment
home/o	the same - r
integument, integumentary system	organ system that covers the body; skin is the main orgain w/i the system;
r- integument	covering the body
lymph	clear fluid collected from body tissues and transported by lymph vessells to the venous circulation; r- lymph,lymphatic system
atic	pertaining to
nervous system	brain, spinal cord, nerves, and sensory receptors, funct: rapidly coordinates body functions and enables learning and memory
nerv	nerve -r
respiration	process of breathing; exchange of carbon dioxide and oxygen
respir	to breathe -r
atory	pertaining to
skeleton	the bony framework of the body
skelet	skeleton -r
urinary system	removes waste from blood, maintains water and electrolyte balance, stores and transports urine; ureters, urethra, urinary bladder, kidneys
urin	urine -r
biopsy	removing tissue from a living person for lab examination
bi	life - r
opsy	to view -s
carcinoma	a malignant and invasive epithelial tumor
carcin	cancer -r
oma	tumor, mass -s
cryosurgery	use of liquid nitrogen or argon gas in a probe to freeze and kill abnormal tissue
cryo	icy cold -r
surg	operate-r
ery	process of -s
cutaneus	pertaining to the skin
cutan/e	skin
dermatology	med specialty concerned w/disorders of the skin
dermat/o	skin
etiology	the study of the causes of a disease
eti/o	cause
excrete	to pass waste products of metabolism out of the body
crete	separate - r
ex	out of, away from -p
ion	action -s
flora	the population of microorganisms covering the exterior and interior surfaces of healthy animals; (latin) flower

prognosis	forecast of the probable future course and outcome of a disease
gnosis	knowledge -r
pro	projecting forward -p
squamous cell	flat, scale-like epithelial cell;(latin) scaly
secrete	to produce a chemical substance in a cell and release it from the cell
secret	produce -r
synthesis	the process of building a compound from different elements
thesis	to organize, arrange -r
syn	together -p
synthetic	built up or put together from simpler compounds
vasoconstriction	reduction in diameter of a blood vessel
vas/o	blood vessel
constrict	narrow -r
dilat	widen, open up -r
vasodilation	increase in diameter of a blood vessel
adipose	containing fat
adip	fat-r
ose	full of -s
analgesic	substance that reduces or relieves the response to pain w/o prod loss of consciousness
alges	sensation of pain-r
an	without -p
dandruff	scales in hair from shedding of the epidermis
dermis	connective tissue layer of the skin beneath the epidermis; middle of 3 layers of skin
derm	skin -r
epidermis	top layer of skin
follicle	spherical mass of cells containing a cavit or a small cul-de-sac; such as hair follicles; (latin) small sac
hypodermis	(subcutaneus) below the dermis, 3rd layer of skin, deepest layer
intradermal	within the epidermis (top layer of skin)
intramuscular	with the muscle
IM	intramuscular
muscul	muscle - r
keratin	protein present in skin, hair, and nails
kerat	hard protein -r
melanin	black pigment found in skin, hair, and the retina
melan	black pigment -r
in	substance -s
sebaceous glands	located in the dermis that open into hair follicles and secrete a waxy fluid called sebum
sebum	waxy secretion of the sebaceous glands
sebac/e	wax
subcutaneus	below the skin; same as hypodermic; 3rd layer of skin, deepest
cutan/e	skin-r
sub	below -p
transdermal	going across or through skin
trans	across, through -p
ultraviolet	light rays at a higher frequency than the violet end of the spectrum
ultra	beyond -p
violet	violet, bluish-purple -r

wheal	hives, small, itchy swelling of the skin; However, wheals raised by an injection do not itch
allergen	substance prod a hypersensitivity (allergic) reaction
gen	produce -s
all	strange, other -r
erg	work, activity -r
atophy	state of hypersensitivity to an allergen - allergic
dermatitis	inflammation of the skin
dermat	skin -r
eczema	inflammatory skin disease, often with a serous discharge; (Greek) to boil or ferment
eczem/a	eczema -r/cf
excoriate	to scratch
cori	skin -r
ex	away from - p
ate	pertaining to -s
pruritis	itching
pruit	itch
anti	against -p
rash	skin eruption
seborrhea	excessive amount of sebum
seb/o	sebum -r
rrhea	flow -s
sebum	waxy secretion of the sebaceous glands
stasis	stagnation in the flow of any body fluid; (greek) stying in one place;
vesicle	small sac containing liquid (eg. a blister) latin-blister
decubitus ulcer	sore caused by lying down for long periods of time
cubitus	lying down -r
ulcer	sore -r
de	from -p
herpes zoster	shingles; painful eruption of vesicles that follows a nerve root on one side of the body; (greek) to creep or spread
macule	small, flat spot or patch on the skin; (latin) spot
malignant	tumor that invades surrounding tissues and metastasizes to distant organs
malign	harmful, bad -r
ancy	state of -s
ant	forming, pertaining to -s
melanin	black pigment found in skin, hair, and retina
melan	black pigment -r
oma	tumor, mass -s
metastasis	spread of a disease from one part of the body to another
stasis	stagnate, stay in one place -r
meta	beyond, subsequent to -p
ize	affect in a specific way -s
stat	stationary -r
nevus nevi (pl)	congenital lesion of the skin; (latin) mole, birthmark
papillomavirus	causes warts and is associated with cancer
papill/o	papilla, pimple -r
oma	mass, tumor - s
virus	(latin) poison

papule	small, circumscribed elevation of the skin; (latin) pimple
verruca	wart casued by a virus (latin) wart
CA	cancer
TB	tuberculosis
SQ	subcutaneous
UV	ultraviolet
staphylococcus aurus	most common bacterium to invade the skin
candida	yeastlike fungus
candidiasis	infection with yeastlike fungus
candid	candida -r
albicans	white
candida albicans	thrush; the most common form of candida; can prod recurrent infections of the skin, nails, and mucous membranes
carbuncle	infection of many hair follicles in asmall area, often on the back of the neck; ingrown hair
cellulitis	inflammation of subcutaneous connective tissue
cellul	cell
fungus fungi (pl)	general term used to describe yeasts and molds
impetigo	infection of the skin prod thick, yellow crusts
infection	invasion of the body by disease-prod microorganisms
infect	internal invasion, infection -r
infectious	capable of being transmitted; a disease caused by the action of a microorganism
infestation	act of being invaded on the skin by a troublesome other species, such as a parasite
infest	invade -r
louse lice (pl)	parasitic insect
mucocutaneous	junction of skin and mucous membrane; (eg. the lips)
muc/o	mucous membrane
cutan/e	skin
ous	pertaining to
necrotizing fasciitis	inflammation of fascia prod deat of the tissue
necr/o	death
fasc/i	fascia (skin)
tiz	pertaining to
ing	quality of -s
parasite	an organism that attaches itself to, lives on or in, and derives its nutrition from another species
parasit	parasite -r (greek) guest
pediculosis	an infection with lice
pedicul	louse -r
osis	abnormal condition
scabies	skin disease prod by mites; (latin) to scratch
tinea	general term for a group of realted skin infections caused by different species of fungi; (latin) worm
toxin	poinsonous substance formed by a cell or organism;
tox	poison -r
ity	state, condition -s
tinea pedis	athlete's foot
tinea capitis	infection of the scalp - ringworm
tinea corporis	ringworm infections of the body's skin and hands

tinea cruris	jock itch; infection of the groin
autoimmune	disease in whihc the body makes antibodies directed against its own tissues; fights self
immune	protected from
auto	self-p
dermatomyositis	inflammation of the skin and muscles
dermat/o	skin
myos	muscle
Kaposi sarcoma	form of skin cancer seen in AIDS patients
psoriasis	rash characterized by reddish, silver-scaled patches; (greek) itch
rosacea	persistent erythematous (redness) of the central face
scleroderma	thickening and hardening of the skin due to new collagen formation
scler/o	hard
derma	skin
symptom	departure from normal health exper by patient
sign	physical evidence of a disease process
systemic lupus	inflammatory connective tissue disease affecting the whole body
system	the body as a whole -r
lupus	(latin) wolf
osus	condition -s
erythemat	redness-r
acne	inflammatory disease of sebaceous glands and hair follicles; (greek) point
androgen	hormone that promotes masculine characteristics
andr/o	male
gen	to produce, create -s
comedo comedones (pl)	too much sebum and too many keratin cells block the hair follicle causing it; a whitehead or blackhead
cyst	greek - sac, bladder; abnormal fluid-filled sac such as gall bladder or urinary bladder, surrounded by a membrane
pustule	small protuberance on the skin containing pus
scar	fibrotic seam that forms when a wound heals; scab
alopecia	hair loss, baldness
cuticle	nonliving epidermis at base of fingernails
matrix	formative portion of a hair, nail, or tooth
onychomycosis	condition of fungus infection in a nail
onych/o	nail
myc	fungus
osis	condition -s
paronychia	infection alongside the nail
para	alongside -p
inflammation	complex of cell and chemical reactions occurring in response to an injury or chemical or biologic agent
flammat	flame
ory	having the funtion of
scald	burn from contact with hot water or steam
shock	sudden physical or mental collapse or circulatory collapse; (german) to clash
allograft	skin graft from another person or cadaver
allo	other-p
graft	transplant
autograft	graft removed from the patient's own skin
auto	self -p

debridement	removal of injured or necrotic (dead) tissue
bride	rubbish -r
de	take away-p
ment	resulting state -s
eschar	burnt, dead tissue lying on top of 3rd degree burns;
heterograft	graft from another species (not human)
hetero	different -p
homograft	skin graft from another person or cadaver; (same as allograft)
homo	same, alike -p
regenerate	reconstitution, rebuilding of a lost part
gener	produce
re	again-p
ation	process-p
ate	composed of-s
xenograft	graft from another species (same as heterograft)
xeno	foreign -p
abdominoplasty	tummy tuck; surgical removal of excess subcutaneous fat from abdominal wall
abdomin/o	abdomen
plasty	surgical repair -s
abrasion	area of skin or mucous membrane that has been scraped off
blepharoplasty	surgical repair of an eyelid
blephar/o	eyelid
clot	mass of fibrin and cells that is prod in a wound
dermabrasion	removal of upper layers of skin by rotary brush
derm	skin
abras	scrape off
granulation	new fibrous tissue formed during wound healing
granul	small grain
ation	process -s
incision	cut or surgical wound
incis	cut into
excis	cut out
excision	surgical removal of part or all of a structure
keloid	raised, irregular, lumpy scar due to excess collagen fiber production during healing of a wound; (greek) stain
laceration	tear or jagged wound of the skin caused by blunt trauma; not a cut
lacer	to tear
lipectomy	surgical removal of adipose tissue
ectomy	surgical excision -s
lip	lipid, fat
lip/o	fat
suct	suck
liposuction	surg removal of adipose tissue using suction
mammoplasty	surg proc to chang the size or shape of the breast
mamm/o	breast
rhinoplasty	surg proc to change the size or shape of the nose
rhin/o	nose
plasty	surgical repair -s
bradycardia	slow heart rate, less than 60 bpm

brady	slow
plasm	to form -r; as suffix - something formed
muscle tissue	func: movement; attached to bones; found in the walls of hollow tubes, organs, and the heart
syn	together, union, association, - p
in -s	substance, chemical compound
cartilage	nonvascular, firm connective tissue found mostly in joints; latin - gristle
chir/o	hand
pract	r - efficient, practical
chiropractic	dx, tx, and prevention of mechanical disorders of the musculoskeletal sys
detoxification	removing poison from a tissue or substance
de	p- from, out of, removal, out of
toxi	r- poison
ligament	band of fibrous tissue connectin 2 structures; latin - band, sheet
muscle	a tissue consisting of cells that can contract
muscul/o	muscle
skelet	skeleton
orthopedic	pert to correction and cure of deformities and diseases of musculoskeletal sys
orth/o	straight -r
ped	child -r
osteopathy	med practice based on maintaining balance of the body
oste/o	bone
pathy	disease -s
path	disease -r
tendon	fibrous band that connects muscle to bone; latin - sinew
number of bones in body	206
amount of blood in body	6 liters
4 components of skeletal sys	bones, cartilage, tendons, ligaments
classification of bones	by shape: long, short - (wrist, ankle, patella) ,flat- (skull,ribs), irregular(vertebrae)
cortex	outer portion of an organ, such as bone
cortic	cortex -r
epiphysis	expanded area at proximal and distal ends of a long bone to prov increased surface area for attachment of ligaments and tendons
physis	r- growth
epi	p - upon, above
haversian canals	vascular canals in bone
marrow	fatty, blood-forming tissue in the cavities of long bones
medulla	central portion of a structure surrounded by cortex, contains marrow; latin - marrow
periosteum	strong membrane surrounding a bone
oste	bone-r
um	structure -r
peri	around -p
epiphyseal plate	growth plate - at ends of long bones allow for growth
achondroplasia	cond w/abnormal, early conversion of cartilage into bone, leading to dwarfism
chondr/o	cartilage
a	without --p

plasia	formation -s
osteogenesis	inherited cond when bone formation is incomplete, leading to fragile, easily broken bones
genesis	formation -s
osteomalacia	soft, flexible bones lacking in calcium - rickets
malacia	abnormal softness -s
osteomyelitis	inflammation of bone tissue; bone marrow infection; caused by bacteria infection like staph
myel	bone marrow
oste/o	bone
osteopenia	decreased calcification of bone, low bone density
penia	deficient -s
osteoporosis	cond in which bones become more porous, brittle, and fragile, more likely to fracture; from loss of bone density
por/o	opening
sis	condition -s
rickets	disease due to Vit D deficiency, prod soft, flexible bones; old english -to twist
sarcoma	malignant tumor orinating in connective tissue
sarc	flesh -r
oma	tumor, mass -s
gen	creation -r
osteogenic sarcoma	malignant tumor originating in bone-producing cells
alignment	having a structure in its corerct postion relative to others
lign	line -r
a	into -p
comminut	break into pieces -r
comminuted fracture	a fx in which bone is broken into pieces
malunion	when 2 bony ends of fx fail to heal together correctly
mal	bad, difficult -p
un	one -r
non	not -p
nonunion	total failure of healing of a fx
osteoblast	a bone-forming cell
blast	immature cell
cyte	cell
osteocyte	a bone-maintaing cell
pathologic fracture	fx occurring at a site already weakened by disease process, such as cancer
path/o	disease
ure	result of - s
fract	to break -r
reduction	restore a structure to its normal position
duct	lead -r
re	backward -p
traction	pulling or dragging force, latin - to pull
external fixation	alignment of fx by immobil bone by plaster casts, splints, traction or external fixators (pins, plates, halo)
external manipulation	bone is pulled from distal end back into algnment through a proc called reduction, often under anesthesia
closed, simple fracture	bone is broken, but skin is not broken
open (comminuted) fracture	a fragment of the fractured bone breaks the skin, or a wound extends to the site of the fx

displaced fracture	fractured bone parts are out of line
complete fracture	a bone is broken into at least 2 fragments
incomplete freacture	fx does not extend completely across the bone; can be hairline, as in a stress fx in the foot when no separation of the 2 fragments
transverse fx	fx is at right angles to the long axis of the bone
impacted fx	fx consists of 1 bone fragment driven into another, resulting in shortening of the limb
spiral fx	fx spirals around the long axis of the bone
oblique fx	fx runs diagonally across the long axis of the bone
linear fx	fx runs parallel to the long axis of the bone
greenstick fx	a partial fx; one side breaks, the other bends (tib/fib and radius/ulna)
compression fx	fx occurs in a vetebra from trauma or pathology, leading to the vertebra being crushed
stress fx	fatigue fx caused by repetitive, local stress on a bone, as occurs in marching or running
axial skeleton	includes: vertebral column, skull, rib cage; protects brain, spinal cord, heart, lungs
vetebral column - how many bones	26
5 regions of vertebral column	cervical -7, thoracic - 12, lumbar -5, sacral -1, coccyx -1
cervical	neck region
cervic	neck -r
coccyx	tailbone, at lowest end of vert column
kyphosis	normal posterior curve of spine that can be exaggerated in disease
kyph	bent, humpback-r
lumbar	region of the back and sides between the ribs and pelvis
sacrum	part of vert column that forms part of the pelvis; latin - sacred
sacr	sacrum -r;
scoliosis	abnormal lateral curvature of vert column
scoli	crooked -r
spine	vertebral column; or short projection from a bone
spin	spine
vertebra, vertebrae (pl)	one of bones of spinal column
vertebr	vertebra -r
whiplash	sym casued by sudden, extesion/flexion of neck
whip	to swing
lash	end of whip
skull - number of bones	22 - 8 cranial, 14 facial
cranium	upper part of skull that encloses and protects brain; greek -skull
crani	skull
ethm	sieve -r
oid	resembling -s
ethmoid	bone that forms the back of the nose and encloses numerous air cells
lacrimal	bone forms part of medial wall of orbit (around eye),
lacrim	tears -r
mandible	lower jaw bone
mandibul	mandible -r
maxilla	upper jaw bone, containing rt and lt maxillary sinuses;
maxilla	maxilla -r
occipital	back of the skull

occipit	back of the head -r
palatine	bone that forms the hard palate and parts of the nose and orbits
palat	palate-r
parietal	2 bones forming the side walls and roof of the cranium
pariet	wall-r
sphenoid	wedge-shaped bone at the base of the skull
sphen	wedge -r
oid	resemble -s
temporal	bone that forms part of the base and sides of the skull
tempor	time; temple-r
mandibul	mandible -r
TMJ - temporomandibular joint	joint between the temporal bone and the mandible (jaw bone joint below ear)
zygoma	bone that forms the prominence of the cheek
zygomat	cheekbone -r
AC	acromioclavicular- lateral end of the scapula, extending over the shoulder joint; at end of clavicle
acromion	joint between acromion and calvicle
acromi	acromion -r
calvicul	clavicle -r
articulate	2 separate bones have formed a joint
articul	joint -r
ation	process-s
articulation	a joint
clavicle	curved bone that forms part of the pectoral girdle
clavicul	clavicle -r
dislocation	completely out of joint
dis	apart, away from -p
locat	place -r
humerus	single bone of upper arm; latin-shoulder
pectoral	pertainint to the chest
pector	chest -r
pectoral girdle	incomplete bony ring tht attaches the upper limb to the axial skeleton; Old eng - girdle
scapula , scapulae (pl)	shoulder blade
subluxation	an incomplete dislocation when some contact between the joint surfaces remains
luxate	dislocate -r
sub	under, below, -p
capitulum	small head or rounded extemity of a bone
capit/u	small head -r
pronat	bend down-r
prone	lying face down on belly
pronation	proc of lying face down on belly position, or turning a hand or foot with volar (palm or sole) surface down
radius	forearm bone on the thumb side; latin - spoke of a wheel
radi	radius -r
supination	proc of lying face upward, or of turning a hand or foot so that the palm or sole is facing up
supinat	bend backward -r
supine	lying face up, flat on back

trochlea	smooth articular surf of bone on which another glides
trochle	pulley -r
ulna	medial and larger bone of forearm; latin - elbow, arm
uln	ulna -r
hinge joint	humrus and ulna - at elbow
gliding joint	humerus and radius
2 articulations of elbow joint	hinge joint - humerus and ulna- allows flexion and extension of elbow; gliding joint between humerus and radius of forearm - allows pronation and supination
arthritis	inflammation of joint(s)
arthr	joint -r
carpus	8 carpal bones of wrist
carp	wrist bones -r
meta	after, subsequent to - p
metacarpals	5 bones between the carpus and fingers
phalanges	finger or toe bones; 14 phalanges of hand- each finger has 3 joints except thumb which has only 2
phalang/e	phalanx, finger or toe
colles fx	fx of distal radius at wrist
eponym	proc or dx with name derived from name of person who discovered it
Heberden node	bony lump on terminal phalanx of fingers in osteoartritis
metacarpophalangeal joint	joints between metacarpal bones and phalanges
osteoarthritis	chronic inflammatory disease of joints
arthr	joint -r
osteo	bone -r
phalanx, phalanges (pl)	one of bones of fingers or toes
rheumatism	pain in various parts of the musculoskeletal sys
rheumat	a flow -
ism	condition -s
rheumatoid arthritis	systemic disease affecting many joints
acetabulum	cup-shaped cavity of hip bone that receives the head of femur to form hip joint; femur goes into hip here
femur	thigh bone
femor	femur -r
illium	large wing shaped bone at the upper and posterior part of pelvis
ischium, ischia (pl)	lower and posterior part of hip bone
ischi	ischium, hip bone -r
pelvis	basin-shaped ring of bones, ligaments, and muscles at the base of the spoine
pelv	pelvis -r
pubis	another name for pubic bone
pub	pubis -r
SI	sacroiliac joint - joint between sacrum and ilium
sacr/o	sacrum -r
ili	illium -r
symphysis	2 bones joined by fibrocartilage; 2 pubic bones; greek - grow together
hip bones - 3 fused together	illium, ischium, pubis
po	by mouth
prn	when necessary
arthrodesis	fixation or stiffening of a joint by surgery

arthr/o	joint -r
desis	to fuse toghether
diastasis	separation of normally joined parts; greek - separation
radi/o	radiation, xrays -r
radiology	study of medical imaging
arthroplasty	surgery to repair, as far as possible, the function of a joint; total replacement of hip joint
plasty	reshaping by surger -s
avascular	to without a blood supply
vascul	blood vessel -r
a	without -p
labrum	cartilage that forms a rim around the socket of the hip joint; latin - lip-shaped
necrosis	pathologice death of cells or tissue; greek -death
necr/o	death -r
prosthesis	artificial part to remedy defect in body; greek - addition
synovial	lubricating
4 ligaments hold knee together	medial collateral ligament, lateral collateral ligament, ACL- anterior cruciate ligament, PCL - posterior cruciate ligament
4 knee joint bones	lower end of femur, flat end of tibia, patella, fibula
collateral	situated at the side; often to bypass an obstruction
later	side
co	together -p
cruciate	re knee - 2 internal ligaments of knee joint cross over each other to form an "x";latin -cross
fibula	smaller of 2 bones of lower leg; latin - clasp or buckle
fibul	fibula -r
meniscus, menisci (pl)	disc of cartilage between bones of a joint, eg the knee joint; greek - crescent
patella, pattellae (pl)	kneecap; thin, circular bone in front of knee joint, embedded in the patellar tendon; laint - small plate
patell	patella -r
tibia	larger bone of lower leg; latin - large shinbone
tibi	tibia -r
arthrocentesis	aspiration of fluid from a joint
arthro/o	joint -r
centesis	puncture -s
arthrography	x-ray of a joint taken after injection of a contrast medium into the joint
graphy	process of recording
arthroscopy	visual exam of interior of a joint
scopy	process of using an instrument to examine visually
arthroscope	endoscope used to exam interior of joint
bursa	closed sac containing synovial fluid
bursitis	inflammation of a bursa
burs	bursa -r
debridement	removal of injured or necrotic tissue
bride	rubbish -r
de	removal, out of -p
hyperflexion	flexion of a limb or part beyond normal limits
hyper	excessive, excess, above, beyond -p
flex	bend-r
meniscectomy	excision (cutting out) of all or part of meniscus (disc of cartilage between the

	bones of a joint, as in knee joint
menisc	crescent, meniscus -r
prepatellar	in front of the patella
patell	patella -r
pre	before, in front of -p
rupture	break or tear of any organ or body part; latin - break, fracture
tendinitis (also spelled tendonitis)	inflammation of a tendon
tendin	tendon -r
bunion	a swelling at the base of the big toe
calcaneus	bone of tarsus (foot) that forms the heel
calcan	calcaneus -r
eal	pertaining to
hallux valgus	deviation of the big toe toward the medial side of the foot (turns out)
hallux	big toe -r
valgus	turn out -r
metatarsus	5 parallel bones of the foot between the tarsus and phalanges
tars	ankle -r
meta	after, subsequent to -p
podiatry	dx and tx of disorders and injuries of foot
pod	foot -r
iatry	treatment
Pott fx	fx of lower end of fibula, often w/fx of tibial malleolus; at ankle
tallus	tarsal bone that articulates w/tibia to form the ankle joint; latin - heel bone
tarsus	collection of 7 bones in foot that form ankle and instep; latin - ankle
tarsal	pert to tarsus
tars	ankle -r
VS	vital signs
SOB	shortness of breath
WNL	within normal limits
MRSA	Methicillin Resistant Stapholococus Aureus- extremely virulent staph infection, can be fatal; use contact isolation - gloves and gown
CDiff	Clostridium Difficile - very contageous diahhrea; contact isolation - gown,gloves
COPD	chronic obstructive pulmonary disease; use Fowlers position
UTI	urinary tract infection
Braden Risk Assessment scale	detailed skin assessment tool
virulence	strength of pathogen
SX	symptoms
dx	diagnosis
VS	vital signs
SOB	shortness of breath
WNL	within normal limits
MRSA	Methicillin Resistant Stapholococus Aureus- extremely virulent staph infection, can be fatal; use contact isolation - gloves and gown
CDiff	Clostridium Difficile - very contageous diahhrea; contact isolation - gown,gloves
HTN	hypertension
COPD	chronic obstructive pulmonary disease; use Fowlers position
UTI	urinary tract infection

Braden Risk Assessment scale	detailed skin assessment tool
virulence	strength of pathogen
SX	symptoms
dx	diagnosis
CVA	coronary vascular accident; stroke
DNRCC	do not resuscitate, comfort care
TIA	trans ischemic attack - mini stroke
HS	hour of sleep; bedtime
FX	fracture
C/O	complains of
A+O	alert and oriented; to : purpose, time, place, person, (A+Ox1, A+Ox2,...)
HTN	hypertension
MI	myocardial infarct - heart attack
CHF	congestive heart failure
AC	before meals
prn	as needed
IDDM	insulent dependent diabetes mellitus
BS	blood sugar, breath sounds, bowel sounds
NIDDM	non-insulent dependent diabetes mellitus
- c	with
tx	treatment
CVA	coronary vascular accident; stroke
TIA	trans ischemic attack - mini stroke
q	every
- p	after
h+P	history and physical
NPO	nothing by mouth
A+O	alert and oriented; to : purpose, time, place, person, (A+Ox1, A+Ox2,...)
SRD	safety reminder device; eg. soft restraint
MI	myocardial infarct - heart attack
AC	before meals
s/p	status post
BS	blood sugar, breath sounds, bowel sounds
- c	with
- s	without
- a	before
- p	after
NPO	nothing by mouth
SRD	safety reminder device; eg. soft restraint
GIB	GI bleed; gastrointestinal bleed
nonblanchable erythema	test for decubitus ulcer- touch reddened area and it does not turn white- if stays red - sign of stage 1 skin break down
atrophy	wasting away or diminished volume of tissue, an organ, or a body part **
hypertrophy	increase in size, but not in number, of an indiv tissue element **
hyper	above, excess, excessive - p
trophy	nourishment -r
a	without -p
contract	draw together or shorten
tract	draw -r

con	with, together - p
fascia	sheet of fibrous connective tissue; latin - a band **
fiber	strand or filament; latin -fiber
multidisciplinary	involving health care providers from omore than one profess
disciplin	instruction -r
multi	many-p
muscle	tissue consisting of cells that can contract
skelet	skeleton -
tone	tension present in resting muscles
voluntary muscle	is under control of the will
volunt	free will-r
functions of skeletal muscle	movement, posture (tone), body heat, respiration, communication
striations	alternating light and dark bands of protein filaments resp for muscle contraction; skeletal muscle - striated muscle
Duchenne muscular dystrophy	cond w/symettrical weakness and wasting of pelvic, shoulder, and proximal limb muscles **
dys	bad, difficult -p
fibromyalgia	pain in muscle fibers **
fibr/o	fiber-r
my	muscle
algia	pain-s
myoglobin	protein of muscle that stores and transports O2
glob	globe-r
in	substance -s
rhabdomyolysis	destruction of muscle to prod myoglobin
lysis	destruction-s
rhabd/o	rod shaped
sprain	wrench or tear in ligament
strain	overstretch or tear in muscle or tendon
tendon	fibrous band that connects muscle to bone
tendin	tendon-r
tendonitis, tendinitis	inflammation of tendon
tenosynovitis	inflamm of tendon and its surrounding synovial sheath
thymectomy	surg remov of thymus gland
thym	thymus gland -r
synov	synovial membrane-r
ten/o	tendon-r
rotator cuff tear	freq injury to shoulder girdle, caused by wear and tear from overuse
insertion	re muscle - attachment of muscle to a more movable part of skeleton, as distinct from the origin
insert	put together -r
ion	action, condition -s
origin	fixed source of a muscle at its attachment to bone
pectoral	pert to chest **
pector	chest -r
pectoral girdle	incomplete bony ring that attaches the upper limb to the axial skeleton **
rotator cuff	part of capsule of the shoulder joint **
rotat	rotate-r
or	one who does-s
cuff	old English-band-r

biceps brachii	muscle of arm that has 2 heads or points of origin on scapula **
brachi/i	of the arm -r
ceps	head -r
bi	two -p
brachialis	muscle that lies underneath biceps and is stronges flexor of forearm
brachi	arm-r
alis	pert to -s
brachioradialis	muscle that helps flex forearm **
brachi/o	arm-r
radi	radius -r
cyst	abnormal fluid-filled sac
deltoid	large, fan-shaped muscle conn scapula and clavicle to humerus
delt	triangle-r
oid	resembling-s
dorsum	back of any part of body, including hand
dors	back-r
ventr	belly-r
ventral	pert to belly or situated nearer to surface of body
ganglion	fluid containing swelling attached to synovial sheath of a tendon
lassissimus dorsi	widest (broadest) muscle in back, the "V" **
dorsi	of the back -r
latiss	wide -r
imus	most-s
stenosis	narrowing of a passage
thenar eminence	fleshy mass at base of thumb
hypothenar eminence	fleshy mass at base of little finger
thenar	palm-r
eminence	latin-stand out
triceps brachii	muscle of arm that has 3 heads or points of origin **
ceps	head-r
brachi/i	of the arm -r
ganglion cyst	fluid filled cyst on back of wrist, result from irritation or inflamm of synovial tendon sheaths
carpal tunnel syndrome CNS)	from inflamm and swelling of overused tendon sheaths; repetitive movements can cause it
abduction	action of moving Away from midline, **
adduction	action of moving toward the midline **
duct	lead-r
ab	away from -p
ad	toward-p
calcaneal tendon	formed from gastronemius and soleus muscles inserted into calcaneus
gastrocnemius	major muscle in back of lower leg (calf)
gastrocnem	calf of leg-r
gluteus	1 of 3 muscles in buttocks
glut	buttocks-r
maximus	gluteus maximus muscle is larges muscle in body, covering large part of each buttock **
medius	gluteus medius muscle is partly covered by gluteus maximus
minimus	gluteus minimus is smallest of gluteal muscles and lies under the gluteus medius

popliteal fossa	hollow at back of knee
poplit/e	ham, back of knee-r
quadriceps femoris	an anterior thigh muscle w/4 heads (origins)
ceps	head-r
orthotic	orthopedic appliance to correct an abnormalty eg. brace **, eg. pins, plates
orthot	correct-r
physical therapy	use of remedial proc to overcome a phys defect** physiotherapy - another term for it
phys	nature-r
iatr	treatment-r
physic	body-r
therapy	systematic tx of disease, dysfunc, or disorder **
contracture	muscle shortening due to spasm or fibrosis **
contract	pull together -r
ure	result of -s
prosthesis	artifical part to remedy a defect in body **
resuscit	revive from apparent death -r **
diaphoresis	sweat, perspiration
diaphor	sweat-r
etic	pert to -s
ECG, EKG,	electrocardiogram; record of elect signals of heart **
electr/o	electricity-r
mediastinum	area between lungs containing the heart, aorta, venae cavae, esophagus
media	middle-p
stin	partition -r
um	structure -s
phleb/o	vein-r
tom	incise, cut -r
tomy	surgical incision-s
aorta	main trunk of systemic arterial sys
endocardium	inside lining of the heart
endo	inside -p
epicardium	outer layer of the heart wall **
epi	above, upon -p
infarct	area of cell death from infarction
farct	area of dead tissue-r
ischemia	lack of blood supply to a tissue
isch	to block, keep back -r
myocardium	all the heart muscle
necrosis	pathologic death of cells or tissue **
necr/o	death - r
pericardium	double layer of membranes surrounding the heart **
pulmonary	pert to lungs and their blood supply **
pulmon	lung-r
atrium	chamber where blood enters heart on both right and left sides
atri	entrance-r
bicuspid	having 2 points; bicuspid heart valve has 2 flaps **
cusp	point-r
id	having a particular quality -s
inter atrial	between atria of the heart

atri	atrium -r
interventricular (IV)	between ventricles of the heart
mitral	shaped like mitre (bishop wears); mitral valve-
4 valves of heart	on right -tricuspid and pulmonary, on left - mitral (bicuspid) and aortic
septum, septa (pl)	thin wall dividing 2 cavities **
tricuspid	having 3 parts; tricuspid heart valve has 3 flaps
ventricle	chamber of heart - pumps blood; also means a cavity in the brain (prod cerebrospinal fluid) **
arrhythmia	cond when heart rhythm is abnormal
atrioventricular (AV)	pert to both the atrium and ventricle
atri	entrance, atrium -r
diastole	dilation of heart cavities, during which they fill w/blood
dysrhythmia	abnormal heart rhythm
murmur	abnormal heart sound heart w/stethoscope when a valve closes or opens abnormally
sinoatrial nodec (SA)	center of modified cardiac muscle fibers in the wall of right atrium that acts as the pacemaker for heart rhythm
sin/o	sinus-r
sinus rhythm	normal (optimal) heart rhythm arising from SA node (sinoatrial)
systole	contraction of the heart muscle
cardiomyopathy	disease of heart muscle, the myocardium
cardioversion	restoration of a normal heart rhythm by electric shock
version	change-s
defibrilation	restoration of uncontrolled twitching of cardiac muscle fibers to normal rhythm
fibrill	small fiber-r
de	from, out of-p
ator	instrument-s
fibrillation	uncontrolled quivering or twitching of the heart muscle
implantable	a device that can be inserted into tissues
pacemaker	device that regulates cardiac electrical
pace	step-r
palpitation	forcible, rapid beat of the heart felt by patient
palpit	throb-r
A-fib	atrial fibrilallation-
v-tach	ventricular tachycardia- rapid heart beat occuring in ventricles
ventricular arrhythmias include	1.PVC's -premature ventricular contractions, 2. v-fib- ventricular fibrillation,
PVC's -premature ventricular contractions-	result when extra impulses arise from a ventricle, 2. v-fib- ventricular fibrillation -occurs when ventricles lose control, quivering instead of pumping
v-fib	ventricular fibrillation -occurs when ventricles lose control, quivering instead of pumping
heart block	occurs when interference in cardiac electrical conduction prevents atria's contraction from coordinating w/ventricles' contractions
palpitations	brief but unpleasant sensations of a rapid or irregular heartbeat; caused by exercise, anxiety, stimulants (caffeine)
AED	automatic external defibrillator- send electric shock to heart in order to stop the heart temporarily so tha a normal contraction rhythm can resume
ICD	implantable cardioverter/defibrillator- sense abnormal rhythms; gives heart small shock to return rhythm to normal
cardiomegaly	enlargement of the heart

megaly	enlargement-s
cor pulmonale	right sided heart failure arising from chronic lung disease
cor	heart-r
ale	pert to -s
endocarditis	inflammation of lining of heart **
exudate	fluid that has passed out of tissue or capillary as result of inflammation or injury
sud	sweat-r
myocarditis	inflammation of heart muscle
pericarditis	inflammation of pericardium, the covering of the heart
prolapse	an organ slips out of its normal position; latin-falling
regurgitate	to flow backward, eg. blood thru a heart valve
gurgit	flood-r
stenosis	narrowing of a canal or passage; eg. of a heart valve
sten/o	narrow-r
tamponade	patholic compression of an organ, such as the heart
tampon	plug-r
ade	a process-s
CO	cardiac output
ASHD	arteriosclerotic heart disease
CAD	coronary heart disease
PNB	pulseless nonbreather
anoxia	without oxygen
an	without-par
arteriosclerosis	hardening of the arteries
arteri/o	artery-r
scler/o	hardness-r
asystole	absense of contractions of the heart
systole/e	contraction-r
atheroma	plaque- fatty deposit in the lining of an artery
ather	porridge, gruel -r
oma	tumor, mass-s
hypovolemic	decreased blood volume in the body
vol	volume-r
occlude	to close, plug, or completely obstruct
substernal	under (behind) the sternum
AHD	atrial septal defect
CHD	congenital heart disease
PDA	patent ductus arteriosus- an open, direct channel between aorta and pulmonary artery in newborn
VSD	ventricular septal defect
coarctation	constriction, stenosis, particularly of aorta
coarct	press together, narrow-r
con	together, with -p
idiopathic	per to disease of unknown etiology
idi/o	unknown-r
syndrome	combin of signs and symptoms assoc w/ a parti disease proc
drome	running-r
HDL	high density lipoprotein - good cholesterol
LDL	low density lipoprotein- bad cholesterol

angiogram	radiograph obtained after injection of radiopaque contrast material into blood vess
angi/o	blood vessel-r
angioplasty	recanalization of blood vessel by surgery
percutaneous	passage thru skin, as by needle puncture
cutan/e	skin-r
per	through-p
stent	wire mesh tube used to keep arteries open
thrombus	clot attached to a diseased blood vessel or heart lining **
thromb	clot-r
ly	break down-r
lysis	dissolve-s **
triglyceride	lipid containing 3 fatty acids
glycer	sweet, glycerol-r
NKA	no known allergies **
artery	blood vessel with oxygenated blood; carries blood away from heart
hemodynamics	science of blood flow thru circulatio
vein	blood vessel carrying blood toward heart
varix, adj- varicose	dilated, tortuous vein
varic	varicosity, dilated, tortuous vein-r
OA	osteoartritis
P	pulse rate
arteriole	small terminal artery leading into capillary network
ole	small-s
capillary	minute blood vessel between arterial and venous systems
capill	hairlike structure-r
palpat	touch, stroke-r
sphygm/o	pulse-r
man/o	pressure-r
steth/o	chest
vena cava	1 of 2 largest veins in body
venule	small vein leading from capillary network
aneurysm	circumscribed dilation of an artery or cardiac chamber
collateral	at the side, often to bypass an obstruction
col	with, together-p
endarterectomy	surg remov of plaque from artery
thromboembolism	piece of detached blood clot (embolus) blocking a distant blood vessel
thromb/o	clot-r
embol	plug-r
thrombophlebitis	inflamm of vein w/clot formation
Hct	hematocrit- percentage of red blood cells in blood
RBC	red blood cell
WBC	white blood cell
anemia	decreased no of red blood cells
an	without-p
colloid	liquid containing suspended particles
plasma	fluid, noncellular part of blood
platelet	(also called thrombocyte)small particle involved in clotting proc
plate	flat-r
let	little, small -s

serum	fluid remaining after removal of blood cells and the formaton of clot
vita	life-r
amin(e)	nitrogen-containing substance -s
functions of blood	1. maintains body's homeostasis, 2. transports nutrients, vit, and minerals, 3. transports waste prod, 4. transports hormones, 5 transports gases- O_2, CO_2, 6. protects from foreign subs- microorganisms+toxins, 7 forms clots
Hgb or Hb	hemoglobin-red pigmented protein; main component of red blood cells
globin	protein-r
agglutinate	stick together to form clumps **
glutin	glue,stick -r
aplastic anemia	cond - bone marrow unable to prod suffic red cells, white cells, and platelets
plas	formation-r
erythrocyte	red blood cell
heme	iron-based part of hemoglobin, carries oxygen
hemolysis	destruction of red blood cells so that hemoglobin is liberated
lyt	destroy-r
hypoxia	below normal level of oxygen in tissues, gases, or blood
pallor	paleness of skin
pernicious anemia (PA)	chronic anemia due to lack of vit B12 **
nici	lethal-r
function of RBC's	transport: oxygen, CO_2, and nitric oxide
agranulocyte	white blood cell w/o granules in cytoplasm
basophil	its granules attract a rosy-red color on staining
granulocyte	a WBC that contains mult small granules in cytoplasm
leukemia	disease when blood is taken over by WBCs and their precursers
leuk	white-r
leukocytosis	excessive number of WBCs
leukopenia	deficient number of WBCs
lymphocyte	small WBC w/large nucleus
monocyte	large WBC w/ single nucleus
mononucleosis	presence of large numbers of specific, diagnostic mononuclear leukocytes
neutrophil	their granuales take up purple stain equally, whterh acid or alkaline
phil	attraction-s
pancytopenia	deficiency of ALL types of blood cells **
pan	all-p
polymorphonuclear	WBC w/multilobed nucleus
morph	shape-r
DIFF	differential white blood count
EBV	Epstein-Barr virus- common virus, member of Herpes family
Ig	immunoglobulin
PMNL	polymorphonuclear leukocyte
leukemia	cancer of blood forming tissues; prod high no of leukocytes
hemostasis	control of bleeding
coagulant	substance that causes clotting
embolus	detached piece of thrombus, mass of bacteria,air, or foreign body that blocks a blood vessel
fibrin	stringy protein fiber; part of blood clot
fibroblast	cell that forms collagen fibers
blast	immature cell-s
hematoma	collection of blood that escaped from vessels into surrounding tissue

hemophilia	inherited disease from defic of clotting factor
stasis	control, stop-s
petechia	pinpoint capillary hemorrhagic spot in skin
prothrombin	protein formed by liver; converted to thrombin in blood clotting mechanism
thromb	blood clot-r
purpura	skin hemorrhages, initially red, then turn purple
thrombocyte, also called platelet	small particle involved in clotting proc
Ab	antibody- protein prod in response to an antigen
antigen	substance capable of triggering an immune response
gen	produce,create-r
ABO	blood group system; type A blood - has only antigen A, type B- has only antigen B, type O-has neither antigen, type AB - has antigen A and B
autologous blood donation	transfusion w/ own blood
Rh	Rhesus
erythroblastosis fetalis	hemolytic disease of newborn (HDN)
Ab	antibody -protein prod in response to an antigen
spleen	vascular lymph organ in LUQ of abdomen
thymus	endocrine gland located in mediastinum
tonsil	mass of lymph tiss on either side of throat @ back of tongue
efferent	moving away from a center
afferent	moving Toward a center
interstitial	pert to spaces between cells in a tissue or organ
Lymphatic system - 3 functions	absorb excess interstitial fluid and return it to bloodstream, remove foreign chemicals, cells, and debris from tissue, 3. absorb dietary lipids from small intestine
adenoid	single mass of lymph tissue in midline at back of throat
aden	gland-r
follicle	spherical mass of cells containing a cavity, eg. hair follicle
immunoglobulin (Ig)	specific protein evoked by an antigen; all antibodies are immunoglobulins
spleen functions	consume bacteria, initiate immune response, consume old, defective erthyrocytes, serve as reservoir
phagocytose	consume
hypersplenism	cond - spleen removes blood components at excessive rate **
inguinal	pert to groin **
lymphadenectomy	surg excis of lymph nodes
lymphaden	lymph node-r
lymphangi	lymphatic vessels-r
Hodgkin	lymphoma- chronic enlargement of lymph nodes spreading to other nodes in orderly way
neoplasm	new growth, benign or malignant tumor
plasm	to form-r
neo	new-p
antecubital	in front of the elbow **
autoimmune	immune rxn directed against person's own tissue
mutation	change in chemistry of a gene
toxin	poisonous subst form by cell or organism
attenuate	weaken the ability of organism to prod disease
attenu	weaken-r
complement	group of proteins in serum- finish off work of antibodies to destroy bacteria

	and other cells
humoral immunity	defense mech from antibodies in blood
humor	fluid-r
anaphylaxis	immediate severe allergic response **
phylac	protect-r
histamine	compound liberated in tissues as result of injury or immune response
incubation	process to dev an infection
incub	lie on, hatch-r
retrovirus	virus w/RNA core
retro	backward-p
tag	touch -r (as in contagious)
endemic	per to disease always present in a community
dem	the people-r
en	in-p
pan	all-p
pandemic	per to disease attacking the population of very large area
nosocomial	acquired w/i a hospital
nos/o	disease-r
com	take care of -r
CA- MRSA	community aquired MRSA- methicillin resistant staphylococcus aureus
SARS	severe acute respiratory syndrome
WNV	West Nile virus
avian influenza	bird flu
alveolus	terminal part of respiratory tract where gas exchange occurs
alveol	air sac -r
bronchus (pl - bronchi)	windpipe; 1 of 2 subdiv. of trachea
cilium (cilia-pl)	hairlike motile projection from surf of cell; latin -eyelash
spirat	breathe -r
olfaction, olfact (r)	sense of smell
oxy	oxygen -r
pharynx (pharyng-r)	tube from back of nose to larnyx (back of throat)
rale	crackle hear thru stethoscope due to fluid in lungs, French - rattle
spir	breathe -r
trachea	air tube from larynx to bronchi
ABG	arterial blood gas
URI	upper respiratory infection
coryza	also called rhinitis- acute inflamm of mucous membrane of nose
congest	r- accumulation of fluid
epistaxis	nosebleed
stax	r-fall in drops
nas	nose -r
palate	roof of mouth, floor of nose
polyp	any mass of tissue that projects outward
rhinitis	acute inflammation of nasal mucosa
rhin	nose -r
sinus	cavity or hollow space in bone or other tissue
CPAP	continuous positive airway pressure
apnea	absence of spontaneous respiration
hypoxemia	low oxygen level in arterial blood
hypoxia	below normal levels of oxygen in tissues, gases, or blood

laryngopharynx	regon of pharynx below the epiglottis that includes the larynx
nasopharynx	reg of pharynx at back of nose and aboe soft palate
pharynx	throat-r
or/o	mouth
polysomnography	test to monitor brain waves, muscle tension, eye movement and oxygen levels in blood as pt sleeps
tonsil	mass of lymph tiss on either side of throat
somn (r)	sleep-r
croup	laryngotracheobronchitis- infection of upper airways in children; with barking cough
epiglottis	leaf shaped plate of cartilage that shuts off the larynx during swallowing
glottis or glott	mouth of windpipe-r
laryngotracheobronchitis	inflamm of larynx, trachea, and bronchi
laryng	larynx -r
papilla	any small projection
stridor	high pitched noise made when respir obstruction in larynx or trachea
pleurisy	inflamm of pleura - membrane covering lungs and lining ribs in thoracic cavity
pleura	membrane covering lungs and lining ribs in thoracic cavity
lobe	subdivision of an organ or other part
bradypnea	slow breathing, less than 10/min
dyspnea	difficulty breathing
eupnea	normal breathing, 12-20 / min
cyanosis	blue discoloration of skin, lips, and nail beds due to low O2 levels in blood
cyan (r)	dark blue -r
eu (r)	normal -r
hemoptysis	blood sputum
ptysis	spit-r
hyperpnea	deeper and more rapid breathing than normal
tachypnea	rapid breathing, over 24/minute
hale (r)	breathe -r
bronchiolitis	inflamm of small bronchioles
bronchiectasis	chronic dilation of bronchi following inflamm disease and obstruction
ectasis (r)	dilation
bulla	bubble like dilated structure
cystic fibrosis	genetic disease w/excessive viscid mucus obstructing passages
emphysema	dilation of respiratory bronchiles and alveoli
physema (r)	blowing
hypercapnia	abnormal increas of CO2 in arterial bloodstream
capn (r)	carbon dioxide
rhonchus	wheezing sound heard on auscultation of lungs; made by air passing thru constricted lumen
viscosity	resistance of fluid to flow
viscos (r)	viscous, sticky
CAO	chronic airway obstruction
CF	cystic fibrosis
adenocarcinoma	cancer arising from glandualr epitheal cells; aden-gland; carcin -cancer
aden (r)	gland
anthrax	severe, malignant infect disease
anthrac (r)	coal

anthracosis	lung disease caused by inhalation of coal dust
aspiration	removal by suction of fluid or gas from a body cavity
atelectasis	collapse of part of lung
atel (r)	incomplete
ectasis (r)	dilatation
empyema	pus in a body cavity, particularly in pleural cavity
hemothorax	blood in pleural cavity
pneumoconiosis	fibrotic lung disease caused by inhalation of different dusts
sarcoidosis	granulomatoous lesion of lungs and other organs
silicosis	fibrotic lung disease from inhaling silica particles
thoracentesis	insertion of needle into pleural cavity to withdraw fluid or air
centesis (r)	to puncture
tubercul (r)	nodule, swelling, TB
AP	anteroposterior
endotracheal	pert to being inside the trachea
spirometer	instrument used to meas respiratory volumes
spir (r)	breathe
thoracotomy	incision thru chest wall
tomography	radiographic image of selected slice of tissue
tom/o (r)	cut, slice, layer
PDT	postural drainage therapy
mucolytic	agent capable of dissolving or liquefying mucus
pneumonectomy	surg removal of a lung
resection	removal of specific part of organ or structure
sect (r)	cut off
tracheotomy	incision into trachea to create tracheostomy
endoscopy	looking inside
septum septa (pl)	a thin wall separting 2 cavities or tissue masses
thrombus	a clot attached to a diseased blood vessel or heart lining
embolus	detached piece of thrombus, a mass of bacteria, quantity of air, or foreign body that blocks a blood vessel
DVT	deep vein thrombosis
lateral collateral ligament	on side of knee, located outside the knee joint; most common ligament damaged in sports injuries
scoiosis	crooked condition of spine
kyphosis	humpbacked condition
autoimmune	immune rxn directed against a person's own tissues
de	without, out of, removal, from
ischemia	lack of blood supply to a tissue
isch	to block,
infarct	area of dead tissue
nosocomial	infection aquired while in the hospital
idiopathic	disease of unknown etiology
sternum	breastbone
scapula	shoulder bone
clavicle	collar bone
derm	skin
SQ, SC	subcutaneous
um	structure
al, ic, ory	pertaining to

lymphedema	tissue swelling due to lyphatic obstruction; differs from regular edema
itis	inflammation, infection
layrnyx	voice box
pharnyx	windpipe
sickle cell anemia	genetic disorder among Afro Amer. RBCs form in sickle shape
pernicious anemia (PA)	chronic anemia due to lack of Vit B12
anemia	red blood cell condition where number of RBCs or amt of hemoglobin in q RBC is reduced
iron deficiency anemia	anemia due to low iron in blood
hemolysis	destruction of red blood cells so hemoblobin is released
lysis	destruction
aplastic anemia	bone marrow is unable to prod sufficient red cells, white cells, and platelets
nici	lethal
agglutinate	to stick together to form clumps
hepat	liver
nephr	kidney
pathy	diseasese
ectomy	surgical removal
tomy	surgical incision
TIA	transient ischemic attack
PVC	premature ventricular contractions
ASD	atrial septal defect
gastroenterologist	specialist stomach and intestines
enterologist	specialist for intestines
lith	stone
rhin	nose
epistaxis	nose bleed
endocrine	gland that prod an internal or hormonal substance and secretes it into bloodstream
exocrine	gland that secretes substances outwardly thru excretory ducts
arthrodesis	surgical fusion of joint
pnea	breathe
apnea	without oxygen; absence of spontaneous respiration
alimentary	pert to digestive tract
aliment	nourishment, food
alimentary canal	digestive tract
an	anus -r
bariatric	tx of obesity
bari	weight -r
atric	treatment -s
esophogus	tube linking pharynx and stomach
gastr	r- stomach
enter	intestine-r
gasteroenterology	med spec of stomach and intestines *
intestin	r- gut, intestine
intestine	digest tube from stomach to anus
laparascopy	exam of contents of abdomen using endoscope
lapar	r-abdomen in general
nutrient	substance in food req for normal physiol funct
nutrit	r-nourishment

bolus	single mass of a substance, Greek-lump
deglutition	act of swallowing
deglutit	r-to swallow
masticate	to chew
mastic	r-chew
peristalsis	waves of alternate contraction and relaxation of intest wall to move food along diges tract *
stalsis	r- constrict
dentine	dense, ivory-like subst located under enamel in tooth
dent	r-tooth
enzyme	protein that induces changes in other substances
zyme	r-enzyme, fermenting
pharynx	r-throat
nas	r- nose
nasopharynx	reion of pharynx at back of nose and above soft pallate
or	r-mouth
papilla	any small projection
parotid	parotid gland is salivary gland beside ear
par	p- beside
ot	r-ear
lingu	r-tongue
mandibul	r-mandible
uvula	fleshy projection of the soft palate
aphthous	canker sores
caries	bacterial destruction of teeth; latin -dry rot
gingiva	tiss surrounding teeth and covering jaw
gigiv	r-gum
halit	r-breath
odont	r-tooth
pyorrhea	purulent discharge
py	r-pus
thrush	infection with candida albicans; occuring anywhere in mouth
dysphagia	difficulty swallowing
phagia	r-swallowing
hernia	rupture; protrusion of structure thru tiss that normally contains it
hiatus	opening thru a structure
hiat	r-opening
postprandial	following a meal
prand	r-breakfast
reflux	backward flow
flux	r-flow
re	p-back
sphincter	band of muscle that encircles an opening, when it contracts the opening squeezes closed; forms a 1 way valve
varic	r- dilated, tortuous vein
chyme	semifluid, partially digested food passed from stomach into duodenum
duoden	r-twelve
gastrin	homrone secreted in stomach stim secretion of HCl and increases gastric motility
HCl - hydrochloric acid	acid of gastric juice

chlor	r-green
intrinsic factor	makes absorption of vit B12 happen
intrins	r- on the inside
factir	r- maker
pepsinogen	converted by HCl in stomach to pepsin
pepsin	enzyme prod by stomach that breaks down protein
pylorus	exit area of stomach
phlor	r- gate, pylorus
anorexia	without appetite
orex	r- appetite
dyspepsia	upset stomach
peps	r-digestion
gastritis	inflamm of lining of stomach
ileum	3rd portion of small intestine
ile	r-ileum
cec	r-cecum
cecum	blind pouch that is 1st part of large intestine
jejunum	segement of small intestine between duodenum and ileum
jejun	r-jejunum
peptic	relating to stomach and duodenum
pept	r- digest
perforat	r- bore through
perforation	hole thru wall of a structure
stricture	narrowing of a tube
bile	fluid secreted by liver into duodenum
bilirubin	bile pigment formed in liver from hemoglobin
cirrhosis	extensive fibrotic liver disease *
cirrh	r-yellow
glycogen	body's prin carb reserve, stored in liver and skeletal muscle
glyc	r- sugar, glycogen
hepat	r - liver
jaundice	yellow staining of tissues w/bile pigments, including bilirubin
liver	body's largest organ,in RUQ abdomen
gnosis	r- knowledge
cholecystitis	inflamm of gallbladder
chol	r-bile
cyst	r- bladder
choledocholithisis	presence of gallstone in common bile duct
cholelithiasis	cond of having gallstones
lith	r-stone
endocrine	gland that pro internal or hormonal subst and secretes it into bllod;
exocrine	gland that secretes sust outwardly thru excretory ducts
endo	p - within, inside
exo	p- outward, outside
gall	r-bitter
gallstone	hard mass of cholseterol, calcium, and billirubin that can be formed in gb and bile duct
glucogen	hormone that mobilizes glucose from body storage
gluc	r-glucose, sugar
agon	r- to fight

insulin	pancreatic hormone that suppresses blood glucose levels and transports glucose into cells
insul	r-island
pancreas	only gland that is both an endocrine and exocrine gland; secretes digestive juices and the hormones insulin and glucagon
celiac disease	caused by sensitivity to gluten
celi	r-abdomen
ease	r- normal function
dia	p-complete
endoscope	general term for a scope to examine colon; specific name for organ used to examine- eg. gastroscope - endoscope to examine stomach
portal vein	carries blood from intestines to liver
villus, villi (pl)	thin, hairlike projection, particularly of mucous membrane lining a cavity
amin	r- nitrogen containing
chyle	milky fluid that results from digestion and absorption of fats in small intestine
emuls	r- suspend in liquid
lacteal	llyph vessel carries chyle away from intestine
lipase	enzyme that breaks down fat
lip	r-fat
ase	s- enzyme
constip	r-press together
Crohn disease	narrowing and thickening of terminal small bowel
enter	r- intestine
dysentery	disease w/diarrhea, bowel spasms, fever, and dehydration
entery	r- condition of intestine
lact	r- milk
sigmoid	simoid colon is shaped like "s"
IBS	irritable bowel syndrome
diverticulum	pouchlike opening or sac from tubualr structure (eg intestine)
fissure	deep furrow or cleft
hemorrhoid	dilated rectal vein prod painful anal swelling
intussusception	slipping of 1 part of bowel inside another to cause obstruction
intus	p- within
suscept	r- to take up
melena	passage of black, tarry stools
occult blood	blood that can't be seen in stool but is pos on feal occult blood test
Hemoccult test	fecal occult blood test
periton	r- stretch over
polyp	mass of tissue that projects into lumen of bowel
proctitis	inflamm of lining of rectum
proct	r - rectum
proctologist	surg spe in disease of anus and rectum
anastomosis	surgicqally made union between 2 tubular structures
ostomy	artificial opening into a tubular structure; end of bowel opens into skin at a stoma; illeostomy, colostomy
stomy	s- new opening
stoma	surgical artificial opening
colostomy	artificial opening from colon to outside of body
ileostomy	artificial opening from ileum to outside of body
gastric	related to the stomach **

gastr	r- stomach *
enter	r-intestine *
gasteroenterology	med specialty of stomach and intestines *
laparoscopy	examination of contents of abdomen using an endoscope *
laparoscope	instrument (endoscope) used for viewing abdominal contents *
laparotomy	incision of intestinal wall
cholecystectomy	surgical removal of gallbladder (cyst-gb)
laparoscopic appendectomy	removal of appendix by endoscope * (look up)
laparoscopic cholesectomy	surgical removal of gallbladder by laparoscope/endoscope
masticate	to chew *
mastic	r- chew
peristalsis	waves of alternate contraction and relaxation of intestinal wall to move food along digestive tract: feeling you have to have BM *
stalsis	r- constrict
peri	p - around
nasopharynx	region of pharynx (windpipe) at back of nose and above soft palate *
oral	pert to mouth
or (os)	r-mouth
palate	roof of the mouth , anterior 2/3 is hard palate, posterior is soft palate *
tongue	mobile muscle mass in the mouth; has the taste buds *
uvula	fleshy projection of the soft palate
saliv	r- saliva
canker sore	aphthous ulcer, erosion of mucous membrane lining the mouth *
cold sore	fever blister, recurrent ulcer of lips, lining of mouth and gums due to infection with herpes simplex virus type 1 (HSV-1) *
caries	bad cavity; bacterial destruction of teeth
gingivitis	inflammation of gums*
gingiv	r- gums
thrush	infection w/Candida albicans; yeast infection/fungus in mouth *
pyorrhea	purulent discharge (pus)
py	r-pus
rrhea	r-flow
asymptomatic	w/o symptoms or abnormalities
symptomat	r-symptom
dysphagia	difficulty swallowing *
phagia	r-swallowing
esophagitis	inflammation of lining of esophagus *
esophag	r- esophagus
hiatal	pert to hiatus (eg. hiatal hernia)
hiatus	opening through a structure
herni	r- hernia
reflux	backward flow
sphincter	band of muscle that encircles an opening: when it contracts, the opening squeezes closed *
GERD	gastroesophageal reflux disease- reflux (regurgitation) of stomach's acid contents into esophagus
esophageal varices	dilated, tortuous veins in esohagus- bleed - can cause death
varices (sing-varix)	dilated, tortuous veins (varicose)
duodenal	pert to duodenum - 1st part of small intestine; 9-12 in long

duoden	r-twelve
chlor	r-green
pylor	r- pylorus, gate *
pylorus	exit area of stomach
chyme	semifluid, partially digested food passed from stomach into duodenum
gastrin	hormone secreted in stomach tath stim secretion of HCl and increases gastric motility
HCl	acid of gastric juice
intrinsic factor	makes absorption of vit B12 happen
mucus	sticky secretion o f cells in mucous membranes
gastroesophageal	pert to stomach and esophagus
anorexia	w/o appetite, an aversin to food
orex	r- appetite
perforation	hole thu wall of a structure
stricture	narrowing of a tube *
perforat	r- bore through
dyspepsia	upset stomach, epigastric pain, nausea, gas
peps	r- digestion
ileum	3rd portion of small intestine
jejenum	segement of small intestine between duodenum and ileum
NSAID	nonsteroidal anti-inflammatory drug
gastritis	inflammation of stomach lining; prod symp of epigastric pain, feeling of fullness, nausea, occasional bleeding
peptic ulcer	(pert to stomach and duodenum) in stomach and duodenum when mucosal lining breaks down
cecum	blind pouch that is 1st part of large intestine
cec	r- cecum
bile	fluid secreted by liver into duodenum
cirrhosis	extensive fibrotic liver disease
cirrh	r- yellow
glyc	r- glycogen, sugar
jaundice	yellow staining of tissues w/bile pigments, including bilirubin
HAV, HBV, HCV	hepatitus A, B, C virus
cholecystitis	inflammation of gallbladder
chole	r- bile
cyst	r- bladder
cholelithiasis	cond having gallstones (bile stones) *
cholelithotomy	surgical removal of gallstones *
insulin	pancreatic hormone suppresses blood glucose levels and transports glucose into cells
pancreas	lobulated exocrine gland, head is tucked into curve of duodenum, prod insulin
insul	r-island
pancreat	r-pancreas
pancreatitis	inflammation of pancreas, causes difficulty regulating insulin and sugar
CF	cystic fibrosis -
glucagon	homrone that mobilizes glucose from body storage
endoscope	instrument used toexamine interior of tubular or hollow organ * (endoscope - look inside, a generic term for scope to examine)
endoscopy	use of endoscope to perform examination
celi	r- abdomen

dis	p - apart
ease	r- normal function
dia	p- apart
flatulence	excessive gas in stomach/intestines
flatul	r- flatus,excessive gas
flatus	gas expelled thru anus
malabsorption	inadequated GI absorption of nutrients * (causes- ciliac and crons disease)
gluten	insoluble protein in wheat, barley, oats
lipase	enzyme that breaks down food *
amino acid	basic building blocks of protein
lacteal	lymph vessel carries chyle away from intestine
lact	r-milk
emuls	r- suspend in a liquid
gastroenteritis	inflammatino of stomach and intestines; stomach flu *
crohn disease	narrowing and thickening of terminal samll bowell
ileus	intestinal obstruction *
anus	terminal end of digestivve tract *
appendectomhy	surg removal of appendix
appendic	r- appendix
colon	large intestine, expanding from cecum to rectum *
rectum	terminal part of colon from sigmoid to anal canal (inside) *
diverticulum, pl- diverticula	puchlike opening or sac from tubular structure (eg intestine) *
fissure	deep furrow or cleft
intussusception	slipping of 1 part of bowel inside another to cause obstruction; telecoping **
intus	r- within
suscept	r- to take up
polyp	mass of tissue that projects into lume of bowel *
proctitis	inflammation of linig of rectum *
proct	r- rectum, anus *
IBS	irritable bowel syndrome
anastomosis	surgically made union between 2 tubular structures *
anastom	r- provide a mouth
colostomy	artificial opening from colon to outside of body
ileostomy	artificial opening from ileum to outside of body
stoma	artificial opening
ostomy	artificail opening into a tubular structure
EEG	electro encephalogram - record of electrical activity of brain *
encephal	r- brain
epilepsy	chronic bran disorder due to paroxysmal excessive neuronal discharges (seizures) *
epilept	r- seizure *
seizure types	gran mal, petit mal, febrile
synapse	junction between 2 nerve cells, or a nerve fiber and its target cell, where electrical impulses are transmitted between cells
afferent	moving Toward a center
dopamine	neurotransmitter in some specific small areas of the brain
glia	connective tissue that holds a structure together
myel	r- spinal cord
myelin	material of sheat around axon of a nerve

neurotransmitter	chemical agent that relays messages from 1 nerve cell to next
sympathetic nervous system	1 of 2 division of autonomic nerv sys operating at unconscious level
parasympathetic nervous system	1 of 2 div of autonomic nerv sys, calms the body, slows down heartbeat, stimulates digestion
autonomic nervous system	self gov visceral motor div of peripheral nerv sys
hypothalamus	* endocrine gland in floor and wall of 3rd ventricle of Brain
cerebrum	cerebral hemispheres
meninges	3 layered covering of the brain and spinal cord *
meningitis	* inflammation of meninges, bacterial or viral; vaccination available !
pia mater	delicate inner layer of meninges
Alzheihmer disease	form of dementia; nvervecells inareas of brain assoc w/memory and cognition are replaced by abnormal protein clumps and tangles
dementia	chronic, progressive, irreversible loss of mind's cognitive and intellectual functions
ment	r- mind
de	p- removal, without
stroke (CVA)	acute clinical event caused by impaired cerebral circulation
grand mal seizure	dramatic form of seizue with: loc, eyes roll up, jaw clenched, may stop breathing
petit mal	seizures of children 5-10; stares vacantly for few seconds
febrile seizure	triggered by fever in infants and toddlers 6 mos - 5 yrs, few dev epilepsy
tic	* sudden, involuntary, repeated contraction of muscles
tonic	state of muscular contraction *
Tourette syndrome	* disorder of multiple motor and vocal tics
aneurism	small, dilation of arter or cardiac chamber
encephalitis	* inflammation of brain cells and tissues; brain swelling causes tissue damage
migraine	severe ha,
mi	p- half, derivied from hemi
graine	r- head pain
syncope	fainting; temporary loc and postural tone due to diminshed cerebral blood flow
alges	r- sensation of pain
concussion	* mild brain injury; brain bruise
concuss	r- shake or jar
countercoup	injujry to brain at point directly opposite point of contact
demyelination	* proc of losing myelin sheat of nerve fiber
esthes	r- sensation
VEP	visual evoked potential
neuropathy	* any disorder of nervous sys
paralyze	make incapable of movement
lyze	r- destroy
lysis	r- destruction
paresis	partial paralysis; weakness r-weakness
poliomyelitis	inflamm of gray matter of spinal cord, leading to paralsis of limbs and muscles of Respiration
polio	r- gray matter
myel	r- spinal cord
drome	r- running
ataxia	* inability to coordinate muscle activity leading to jerky movements

tax	r- coordination
paraplegia	paralysis of Both legs
pleg	r- paralysis
quadriplegia	paralysis of all 4 limbs
spina bifida	failure of one or more vertebral arches to close during fetal development
teratogen	agent that produces fetal deformities (eg. thalidomide)
terat	r- malformed fetus, monster
anxiety	distress and dread caused by fear
bipolar disorder	modd disorder with alternating periods of depression and mania
mania	mood disorder w/hperactivity, irritability, and rapid speech
man	r- frenzy
psychosis	disorder causing mental disruption and loss of contact w/reality
paranoia	presence of persecutory delusions
conjunctiva	inner lining of eyelids
cornea	central, transparent part of outer coat of eye covers iris and pupil
lacrimal	pert to tears and tear apparatus
ptosis	cond - upper eyelid is constantly drooped over eye, due to paresis ofmuscle that raises upper lid
conjunctivitis	inflamm of conjunctiva- inner lining of eyelids
nasolacrimal	passage from lacrimal sac to nose
lacrim	r- tear
duct	r- to lead
photophobia	fear of light because it hurts eyes
opthamology	dx and tx of diseases of eye
blepharities	inflammation of eyelid
blephar	r- eyelid *
blepharoptosis	drooping of eyelid
paresis	partial paralysis
contamination	presence of infectious agent on any surface
accomodation	act of adjusting somethng to make it fit the needs
commodat	r- adjust
amblyopia	failure or incomplete dev of pathways of visionto brain; lazy eye *
esotropia	turning eye inward toward nose; cross-eyed
eso	p- inward
exo	p- outward
exotropia	turning eye outward away from nose
ocular	pert to eye
ocul	r- eye
optometrist	skilled in meas of vision, can't treat or pres meds
stabismus	turning eye away from its normal position *
strab	r- squint
ismus	s- take action
iris	colored portion of eye w/pupil in center
dilation	stretching or enlarging an opening or structure
constric	become narrow
strict	r- narrow
lens	transparent refractive struc behind iris
presbyopia	difficulty in nearsighted vision occurring in middle and old age
presby	r- old man
retina	light sensitive innermost layer of eyeball

sclera	white of eye
scler	r- white of eye, hardness *
photoreceptor	cell receives light and converts it into electrical impulses
uvea	middle coat of eyeball, includes iris, ciliary body, choroid
visual acuity	* sharpness and clearness of vision
astigmatism	inability to focus light rays that enter the eye in different planes
stigmat	r- focus
hyperopia	able to see distant objects but unable to see close ** (farsighted)
myopia	able to see close objects but unable to see distant; nearsighted
opia	r- sight
myop	r- to blink
hyper	r- beyond
cataract	complete or partial opacity of lens
glaucoma	increased intraocular pressure
glauc	r- lens opacity
angiography	radiography of vessels after injection of contrast material
laser surgery	use of concentrated, intense narrow beam of electromagnetic radiation for surg
opthalmoscope	instrument for viewing retina
opthalm	r- eye
retinoblastoma	malignant neoplams of primitive retinal cells
retinopathy	* degenerative disease of retina
peripheral vision	ability to see objects as they come into the outer edges of visual field
acetaminophen	analgesic and antipyetic (pain and fever)
acute	sudden onset
chronic	persistent, long-term disease
otitis media	inflamm of middle ear
otologist	med spec in disease of ear
otorhinolaryngologist	EENT -ear, nose, throat med specialist
rhin	r- nose
laryng	larynx- throat
auricle	shell- like external ear
cerumen	ear was
otoscope	instrument to examine ear
ot	r- ear
pinna	auricle - external ear
typan	r- eardrum
adenoid	lymph tissue in midline at back of throat*
aden	r- gland
eustachian tube	* tube connects middle ear to nasopharynx
ossicle	small bone, particularly relat to 3 bones in middle ear
mast	r- breast
stapes	inner (medial) one of 3 ossicles of middle ear, shaped like a stirrup
coryza	acute rhinitis; viral inflammof mucous membrane of nose
myringotomy	incision in typanic membrane
myring	r- tympanic membrane
tympanostomy	surg created new opening in tympanic membrane to allow fluid to drain from middle ear (ear tubes)
tympan	r- eardrum
cochlea	combination of passages; describe inner ear

labyrinth	inner ear
librium	r- balance; equilibrium - equally balanced
otolith	calcium particle in vestibule of inner ear (ear stone)
vestibule	space at entrance to canal
endocrine gland	prod internal or hormonal secretion
crine	r- secrete
hormone	chemical formed in 1 tissue or ogran and carried by blood to stim or inhiit a functin of another tissue or organ
pineal gland	endocrine gland in floor an dwall of 3rd ventricle of brain; secretes feel-good hormone serotonin by day and converts it to melatonin at night
seratonin	feel good hormone; neurotransmitter in CNS and PNS
melatonin	hormone formed by pineal gland helps regulate sleep and wake cycles
hypothalamus	endocrine gland in floor and wall of 3rd ventricle of brain; prod 8 hormones
endocrine system	pituitary gland, pineal gland, thyroid gland, 4 parathyroid glands, thymus, 2 adrenal glands, pancreas
protaglandin	hormone present in many tissues, but first isolated from prostate gland
corticosteroid	hormone prod by adrenal cortex
cortisone	corticosteroid prod in small amounts by adrenal cortex
DI - diabetes insipius	excretion of large amounts of dilute urine as result of inadequate antidiuretic hormone prod
hydrocortisone	potent glucocorticoidw/ antiinflammatory properties
tropin	s- stimulation
thymus	endocrine gland in mediastinum
thyroid	endocrine gland in neck
exophthalmos	protrusion of eyeball
opthalmos	r- eye
hyperparathyroidism	excessive levels of parathyroid hormone;
hypoparathyroidism	deficient levels of parathyroid hormone;
hyperpyrexia	extremely high body temperature or fever
hyperthyroidism	excessive prod of thryroid hormone; increases body metabolism, including protruding eyes, tachycardia, htn, diaphoresis, treamor, anxiety, diarrhea, weight loss
hypothyroidism	deficient prod of thyroid hormone; decreases body's metabolism
adrenal gland	endocrine gland o upper pole of each kikney
nephr	r- kidney
idiopathic	pert to disease of unknown origin
idi	r-unknown
glucose	final product of carbohydrate digestion; main sugar in blood
insulin	hormone produced by islet cells of pancreas
islets of Langerhans	areas of pancreatic cells that prod insulin and glycagon
diabetes mellitus	metabolic syndrome caused by absolute or relative insulin deficiency and/or ineffectiveness
IDDM	insuline dependent diabetes mellitus; type 1 diabetes,
NIDDM	non-insuline dependent diabetes mellitus, type 2 diabetes
hyperglycemia	high blood glucose level, over 110
hypoglycemia	low blood glucose level; under 70
paresthesia	abnormal sensation - tingling, numbness, burning, prickling
esthes	r- sensation
polydipsia	excessive thirst
dips	r- thirst
polyphagia	excessive eating

polyuria	excessive production of urine
retinopathy	degenerative disease of retina
ketoacidosis	excessive ketones in blood making it acid
metabolic acidosis	decreased pH in blood and body tissues as result of upset metabolism (under 7.35)
p	chemical formed in uncontrolled diabetes or in starvation

Nursing Medical Terminology

Word Search

Med Terminol Word Search Puzzle

```
I T I S H L H S N L Y M O T C E T S Y C E L O H C P O R T E R C H A I
A C H O N D R O P L A S I A V F I B P N M A T S N I C A T E D F Z I X N
S R S I N A R C E S T D O T S E Y S R U T J O X J U E Y K D H C R T V R
U E R U T C I R T S A T E H E O R R U T B O G M L R C F L L K B O Y G S U
S J Z U E G L T E M N Y C E P E B H O P T O G M K R C I W O D Z Y G A P S
C E K A H Y K I M Y C E N Q Y G L M G C R Y O S U R G E R Y I E L A H T O
E N B D E C I K A O N G L M A P A E N P F C L R I S H C N C E I M O N Y P
P B L M C J C V G P T Y H N P O I E H U H X F U O U T A C U N N Y L U P A
T L E M J O I V H J M I J L H O E M Y O P I A P N J Y E Y G O N G L E A R
K E G M C J V R A R E L C S O I R E T R A Z U U N H K R H V Z A L G O E T E
H Z I O B R O L O G Y S I T E N D I N C A N V P P R G V E N U L E F Y C H
C A W B R A E L C S O I R E T N D I P I G L O T T I S T A M I C R O C Y T
T S I O R E L C S O I R E T R A Z U U N H K R H V E R O C Y T E U H A F A
E T R A H C S E T N S E G L O T T I S T A M I C R O C Y T E U H A P F R E
H R A H C S E T N S E P I G L O T T I S T A M I C R O C Y T E U H A T
```

☐ STRICTURE	☐ PNEA	☐ NEUROLOGY
☐ CRYOSURGERY	☐ OCCIPITAL	☐ ARRHYTHMIAS
☐ PATH	☐ PAPILL/O	☐ ATOPHY
☐ DEMENTIA	☐ SPHENOID	☐ PNEUMOTHORAX
☐ LEUKEMIA	☐ ARTERIOSCLEROSIS	☐ EPILEPT
☐ BRACHI/O	☐ NUCLEOLUS	☐ ETIOLOGY
☐ TOMOGRAPHY	☐ HYPOGASTRIC	☐ HEME
☐ GLOB	☐ PLASTY	☐ INFUSION
☐ ACHONDROPLASIA	☐ LENS	☐ TENDIN
☐ CHOLECYSTECTOMY	☐ V-FIB	☐ ESCHAR
☐ ITIS	☐ GRANUL	☐ SUSCEPT
☐ CYT/O	☐ PLEURISY	☐ EPIGLOTTIS
☐ RHIN	☐ ECTASIS (R)	☐ PAPULE
☐ ANCY	☐ MICROCYTE	☐ MASTICATE
☐ VENULE	☐ RETRO	☐ MYOPIA
☐ OSTEOCYTE	☐ LYMPH	☐ THERAPY
☐ SYSTOLE/E	☐ AGON	

Med Terminol Word Search Puzzle

```
T O D N E W M Y H Y L H P I N S U L I N A V B P H A L A N G E Z X W A
U O E O J X S L E K S T M H K S G J X O T O V E K T A S T S O M E H C
J T H U Y Y O J M F I A U E A Y R A C J I L W P O V P C U O A U R I D
L R E C P D U S A T R R I T R G G O S N O U Z M Y E A O S E L V B P U
S K C R I N I W T L U R D Y I L I Y D T N N H N Y G R L U N V B G L A
B O C C U K E I O F R H R C V M I A Z J R T Q W P G I I M A E E A A S
C N A O V S Y A M G C Y A O S Z W X T H E I Z D R N C O A T O R S S F
V L U L L E C D A I A T C R P O Q N J E J U N P S K C S L U L E T H A
W D K Y A B M S Q R E H I C Y P A T E L L F I U D Z I I A L C V R S R
L Y M P H V T G R T N M R I O N I M O D B A L T H R U S H B L I C R U
V R A L U C O R F A I I E M G T K A E N A Y L D A R B X O T U B R C E
G Q T U Y H B M A E T A P I Y K A Q B E X O C R I N E P O S T R T M L
M A C R O C Y T A L D M L B R O N C H I E C T A S I S T P A I I S B P
C O L L A T E R A L H A M S I S O B A N A H R E P I L H Y S I S X Y M
C O K H E C N E N I M E R A N T H T O P Y H E K A I L I H P O M E H T
```

- ☐ ATRI
- ☐ HEART BLOCK
- ☐ LAPAR
- ☐ WHIPLASH
- ☐ ARRHYTHMIA
- ☐ COCCYX
- ☐ SUBCUTANEUS
- ☐ OCULAR
- ☐ COLLATERAL
- ☐ ATRI
- ☐ ANABOLISM
- ☐ BRONCHIECTASIS
- ☐ INSULIN
- ☐ ABDOMIN/O
- ☐ ETHM
- ☐ EPIGASTRIC
- ☐ ALVEOL
- ☐ EXOCRINE
- ☐ ENDO
- ☐ INSUL
- ☐ HEMATOMA
- ☐ BRADYPNEA
- ☐ MALIGNANT
- ☐ GASTRIN
- ☐ HYPOTHALAMUS
- ☐ HYPOTHENAR EMINENCE
- ☐ PHALANG/E
- ☐ DORS
- ☐ MICROCYTE
- ☐ PATELL
- ☐ EPIPHYSIS
- ☐ PERICARDIUM
- ☐ PHAGIA
- ☐ MACROCYTE
- ☐ ATION
- ☐ CELLUL
- ☐ VOLUNT
- ☐ THRUSH
- ☐ TINEA CRURIS
- ☐ PLEURA
- ☐ JEJUN
- ☐ LYMPH
- ☐ HEMOPHILIA
- ☐ UTERUS
- ☐ SCOLIOSIS
- ☐ ACID/O
- ☐ CEREBRUM
- ☐ EUPNEA

Med Terminol Word Search Puzzle

```
S T E N O S K E L E T P J M K G V E O M U S C L E E W Q O T Y C V S P
O C C U L T B L O O D U A I D R A C Y D A R B P L N N J O Y S A A L E
S A O M N Z L B C O L L O I D Z K N C E R V I X E D O G H Q I Q N P P
I R N C I F M L G I I M E D N A P C G D U D F I A O K P T X S F A I T
S T Z S H I G E N C P O R T Z Z B R I L W F F I E T A N S R A T T L I
O E F T R I A P P I A N T I G E N A O N I O D F P R O T F X I F O I C
H R W V N G E H R D R O N Y U M B A G T B G X J N A X G L C H M Y V U
C I C S O L N A U U O L Z N L E N E D A H R N O X C E K O S T N L S L
Y O U U C T E R R S N O I E T N S T I N B H R J O H L X R W I R D U C
S L H I T H Q I I Q Y G Q K R E P L Z U Z Z O R E E F B A M L F L L E
P E R F R A L T T I C I J E A Y F I X R T U H M I A O R O E E D D I R
L U B R K I N I I G H S R R P H H G C N O R H A E L M D E I L E K L C
A D O H G S Y E S I I T L L S Z Z N A I H R Z B D I B L S H L C P I P
V Y P H A I C S A S A N O O T Z Z I L E T T U F H A N H H N I U Y V Y
P S N O I T C N U N N E E E P O O S T E E O M E R I T I S F C T O X Y
```

☐ PYORRHEA
☐ OCCULT BLOOD
☐ PARONYCHIA
☐ FLORA
☐ CHOLELITHIASIS
☐ AURICLE
☐ FERTILIZATION
☐ INTESTIN
☐ TARS
☐ ENDOTRACHEAL
☐ OSTEOMYELITIS
☐ VILLUS, VILLI (PL)
☐ RHIN
☐ INSUL
☐ CERVIX
☐ LASH
☐ CUTAN/E

☐ ARTHROGRAPHY
☐ ANTIGEN
☐ MUSCLE
☐ SPLEEN FUNCTIONS
☐ HYPER
☐ PULMONOLOGIST
☐ CYT/O
☐ PANDEMIC
☐ GANGLION
☐ ARTERIOLE
☐ COLLOID
☐ LIGN
☐ PROTHROMBIN
☐ THROMB
☐ FASCIA
☐ PRURITIS

☐ STEN/O
☐ ULTRA
☐ ANATOMY
☐ BLEPHARITIES
☐ SKELET
☐ FLEX
☐ ORGAN
☐ DIABET
☐ ABDOMIN
☐ ADEN
☐ BRADYCARDIA
☐ TROPIN
☐ PEPTIC ULCER
☐ SHOCK
☐ PSYCHOSIS
☐ CROUP

Med Terminol Word Search Puzzle

```
L Y S I S P A H D I N T R I N S X L W C M E T A S T A S I S N B C I G
I O F V C R C T M T J U S K D Z F N Z M A O M X P Y A A M Q C P M I N
R N J J T C I S O C A Q B Q I P O D F A D M L Z C T H R G A O F U F G
S V T H D I T A T R I K M I T O L S B R R I C S A S T L S O B C N S O
E Y R U S R R L P A F R S I T Z W G I P E T S A S I L P A R T K U A W
M L N I S T O B M Y F O M A X Z W Y T A N H N A N I F P O R O B M M D
D A S O X S C B Y I C O N C U S S I O N E F P I O M E T A M A A A M C
Y H T X V N L A S Y F O L L I C L E N S G S K D Z N C O O I C L T A D
W V Y R S O I G X A R H T N A E L E C T R O O R J F I M K O T B E T S
V D X G I C K O T P E E N A R B M E M L A I V O N Y S M W N U I C I U
W T G D P X U N V A N G I O G R A M I L E R O S D L O C A R R C A O M
D E R M A T O M Y O S I T I S V E L E C T R O O Q S Q Y T B T E A N S
M E N I N G I T I S Y T S A L P O M M A M C M U A L Y T E I X N A L I
Y F F U C R O T A T O R W H I P L A S H M M S C P G F A C T I R S F L
H Y P O G L Y C E M I A E C O N T R A C T C E K D P H A G I A K T V B
```

- FARCT
- AGON
- DERMATOMYOSITIS
- META
- FLORA
- ODONT
- GENER
- INTUS
- SYNOV
- CONSTRIC
- ANGIOGRAM
- MAMMOPLASTY
- ACROMION
- LYSIS
- ALBICANS
- FACTIR
- ACETABULUM
- CONTRACT
- POR/O
- EPIGLOTTIS
- SYNOVIAL MEMBRANE
- ISMUS
- AMINO ACID
- COLD SORE
- GLYC
- INTRINS
- INFLAMMATION
- CONTRACTURE
- BLAST
- CONCUSSION
- FOLLICLE
- DIST
- SYMPTOM
- WHIPLASH
- ELECTR/O
- PRONATION
- PHAGIA
- CORTIC
- ARTHR
- MENINGITIS
- ELECTR/O
- CA- MRSA
- ROTATOR CUFF
- ALLO
- HYPOGLYCEMIA
- METASTASIS
- INTRA
- MATRIX
- ANTHRAX
- ANXIETY

Med Terminol Word Search Puzzle

```
W P S I N O E U M M F O C O L L A G E N Q U T E N W L G V R G P Q N E
X R B R M T M A F R E E T L S B R D Y E H P S M P P H T D U Z A N E N
N O U P H U Z J R R C M I O M T R X E A L T E U N S I M U P B N C U T
Y N K O C V A J R Y A M D O L G D G G E K O V L V A O S T T G C E R E
R E S R Y S T R F F U O O A P I S G M E C Q T S K I P E S U G Y R O R
A K D L Z Z N I C E S R R P E D H H I P E Y A N Y S N I U R C T B P F
H A A U L I D Q U S H O S B R X L L L O H I S P A S K K L E T O I L Z
P O B N U U I B O Q H Q C H I G J J J I N I N T H W L Z K L R P L R D
O R R M N G J T O X B B O E I L D O O I O C Y T E A L X D D O E I H H
S O Z A W U M T O X I N O E L Y O X N L L J R C L O E R I G I I R D G
A S R G W A B D U C T I O N Y P B U E A I K U L N D L L X L B I U U G
N G S E B O M A L A C I A H P B B H S A T I B S A F N E N E X A B R U
A E N I P U S N U C L E O L U S E U G N L C O L O Z A Q N L Y C I R D
S P H E N O I D J P L O T A P E H I T A A S B N A I O O N S M R N R U
G E N E R E X C O R I A T E F F S T I B T R H O T M O M R H T H D Y D
```

☐ HEPAT	☐ ABDUCTION	☐ AGRANULOCYTE
☐ HIST/O	☐ ETHM	☐ CRANIUM
☐ OTOLITH	☐ MUCOSA	☐ SUPINE
☐ CARDIOMEGALY	☐ MEDIA	☐ NUCLE/O
☐ BILIRUBIN	☐ PRONATION	☐ PRONE
☐ SEB/O	☐ THROMBOPHLEBITIS	☐ TENS
☐ OR (OS)	☐ SPHENOID	☐ GENER
☐ BRACHI/I	☐ EXCORIATE	☐ MALACIA
☐ NUCLEOLUS	☐ RHEUMAT	☐ EMULS
☐ DORS	☐ TOXIN	☐ ATION
☐ COLLAGEN	☐ ORIGIN	☐ SIN/O
☐ ALOPECIA	☐ LYMPHADEN	☐ ANABOLISM
☐ RUPTURE	☐ ASYSTOLE	☐ BRACHI/O
☐ NEUROPATHY	☐ CYTE	☐ PERI
☐ FOLLICLE	☐ ENTER	☐ PELVIS
☐ NASOPHARYNX	☐ PANCYTOPENIA	☐ FASCIA
☐ PAPILL/O		

Nursing Medical Terminology

Crosswords

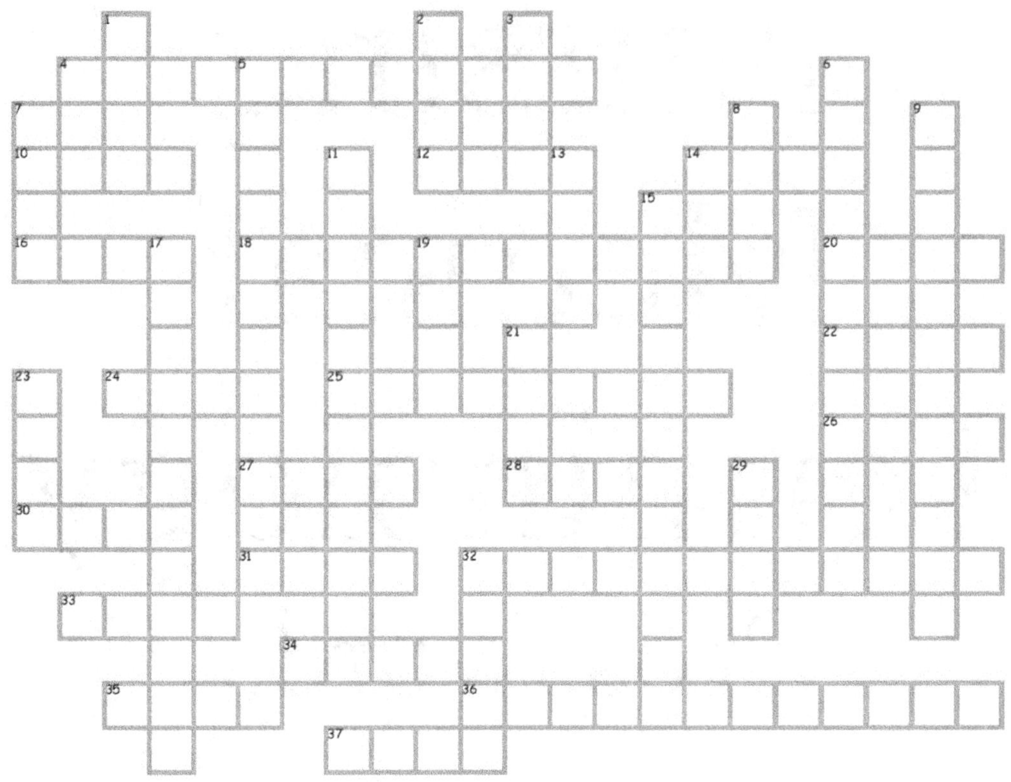

Across

4 organelles that generate, store, and release energy for cell activities
10 pert to -s
12 r- mind
14 triangle-r
16 to block, keep back -r
18 inherited cond when bone formation is incomplete, leading to fragile, easily broken bones
20 instrument-s
22 unknown-r
24 after, subsequent to -p
25 pertaining to the back surface of the body, situated behind
26 pert to mouth
27 ankle -r
28 life-r
30 tension present in resting muscles
31 abnormal fluid-filled sac
32 removal of upper layers of skin by rotary brush
33 Methicillin Resistant Stapholococus Aureus- extremely virulent staph infection, can be fatal; use contact isolation - gloves and gown
34 arteriosclerotic heart disease
35 chronic obstructive pulmonary disease; use Fowlers position
36 complex of cell and chemical reactions occurring in response to an injury or chemical or biologic agent
37 back-r

Down

1 tibia -r
2 insulent dependent diabetes mellitus
3 physical evidence of a disease process
5 dx, tx, and prevention of mechanical disorders of the musculoskeletal sys
6 excessive ketones in blood making it acid
7 radius -r
8 head -r
9 increase in diameter of a blood vessel
11 cond in which bones become more porous, brittle, and fragile, more likely to fracture; from loss of bone density
13 tendon-r
15 soft, flexible bones lacking in calcium - rickets
17 high BP
19 r-mouth
21 pelvis -r
23 lead-r
29 bursa -r
32 to fuse toghether

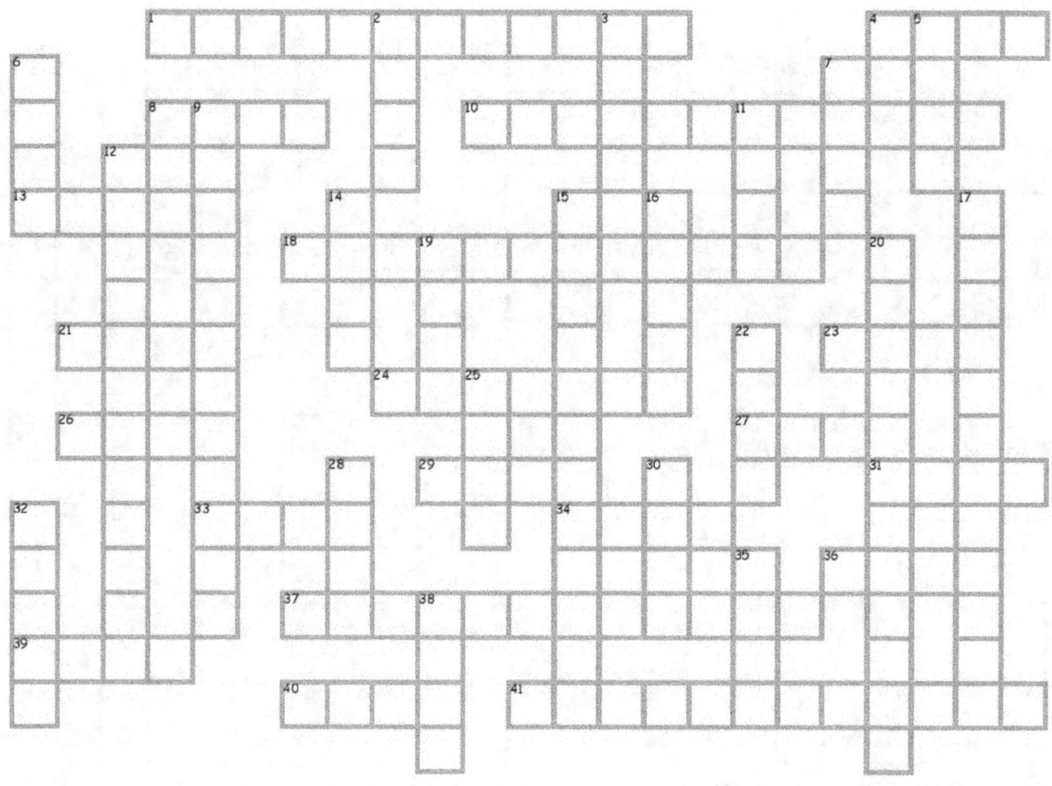

Across

1. inflammation of eyelid
4. blood vessel
8. cause
10. paralysis of all 4 limbs
13. large wing-shaped bone at the upper and posterior part of the pelvis (Latin) groin
18. low blood glucose level; under 70
21. urine -r
23. s - body
24. homrone secreted in stomach stim secretion of HCl and increases gastric motility
26. r- thirst
27. skin eruption
29. iron-based part of hemoglobin, carries oxygen
31. thymus gland -r
33. to view -s
34. nerve -r
36. step-r
37. excessive ketones in blood making it acid
39. same, alike -p
40. stationary-r
41. air in the pleural cavity

Down

2. fat-r
3. within - p
5. pertaining to
6. skin-r
7. skin -r
9. surg created new opening in tympanic membrane to allow fluid to drain from middle ear (ear tubes)
11. p- around
12. pouchlike opening or sac from tubualr structure (eg intestine)
14. r/cf - cell
15. high BP
16. black pigment -r
17. extremely high body temperature or fever
19. r- sight
20. protrusion of eyeball
22. operate-r
25. r- solid
28. s - soluble
30. icy cold -r
32. disease -rdisease -s
32.
35. r/cf -thread
38. r - bone

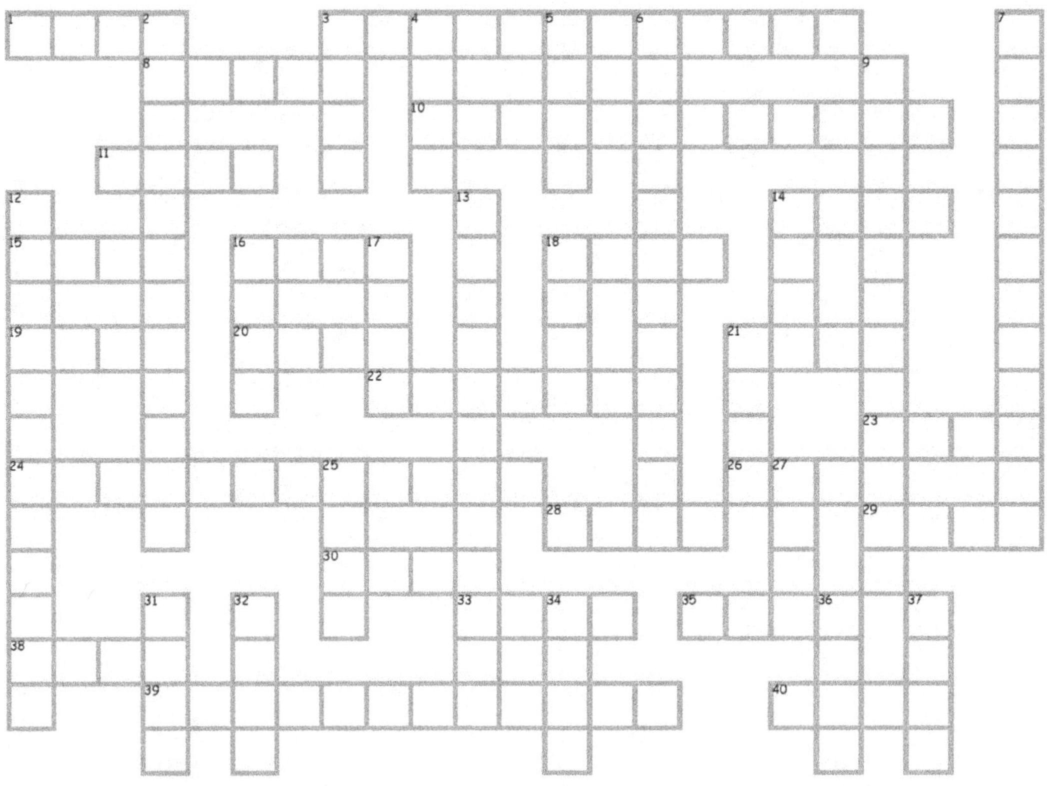

Across

1. medial and larger bone of forearm; latin - elbow, arm
3. air in the pleural cavity
8. greek - sac, bladder; abnormal fluid-filled sac such as gall bladder or urinary bladder, surrounded by a membrane
10. extremely high body temperature or fever
11. r- poison
14. muscle
15. foreign -p
16. mucous membrane
18. bone-r
19. alongside -p
20. lethal-r
21. other-p
22. r- constrict
23. skin
24. low blood glucose level; under 70
26. fibrotic seam that forms when a wound heals; scab
28. inflammatory disease of sebaceous glands and hair follicles; (greek) point
29. s - pertaining to
30. self-p
33. physical evidence of a disease process
35. cell
38. r- sight
39. surg created new opening in tympanic membrane to allow fluid to drain from middle ear (ear tubes)
40. fat

Down

2. act of adjusting somethng to make it fit the needs
3. around -p
4. sieve -r
5. r- appetite
6. high BP
7. passage from lacrimal sac to nose
9. organelles that generate, store, and release energy for cell activities
12. protrusion of eyeball
13. excessive ketones in blood making it acid
14. bone marrow
16. resulting state -s
17. abnormal condition
18. condition -s
21. pert to -s
25. continuous positive airway pressure
27. mass of fibrin and cells that is prod in a wound
31. disease -r
32. same, alike -p
34. globe-r
36. pert to -s
37. instrument-s

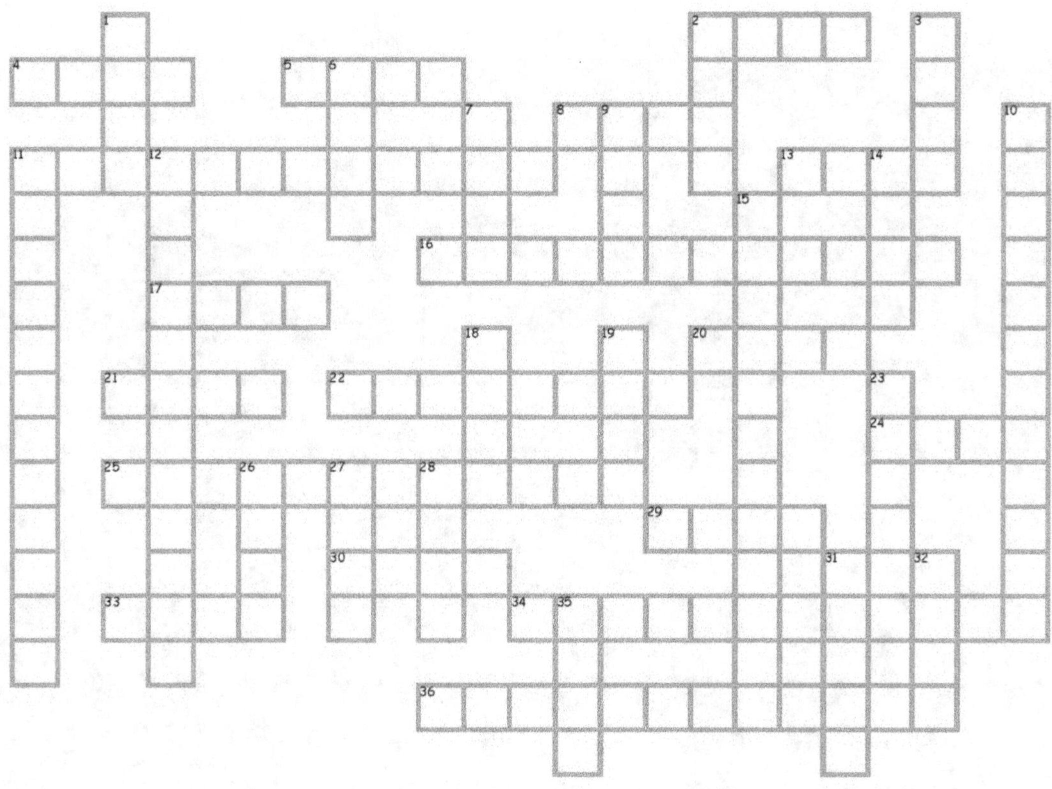

Across

2 blood vessel carrying blood toward heart
4 buttocks-r
5 step-r
8 lethal-r
11 x-ray of a joint taken after injection of a contrast medium into the joint
13 gland-r
16 cond in which bones become more porous, brittle, and fragile, more likely to fracture; from loss of bone density
17 inside -p
20 sinus-r
21 atrial fibrilallation-
22 front surface of the body;
24 partition -r
25 excision (cutting out) of all or part of meniscus (disc of cartilage between the bones of a joint, as in knee joint
29 formation-r
30 p- after
33 back-r
34 increase in diameter of a blood vessel
36 organelles that generate, store, and release energy for cell activities

Down

1 lead-r
2 ventricular fibrillation -occurs when ventricles lose control, quivering instead of pumping
3 nose -r
6 entrance-r
7 nature-r
9 unknown-r
10 high BP
11 surgery to repair, as far as possible, the function of a joint; total replacement of hip joint
12 flexion of a limb or part beyond normal limits
14 pert to -s
15 a joint
18 triangle-r
19 surgical incision-s
23 to block, keep back -r
26 most-s
27 head-r
28 point-r
31 treatment-rtreatment
31
32 life-r
35 instrument-s

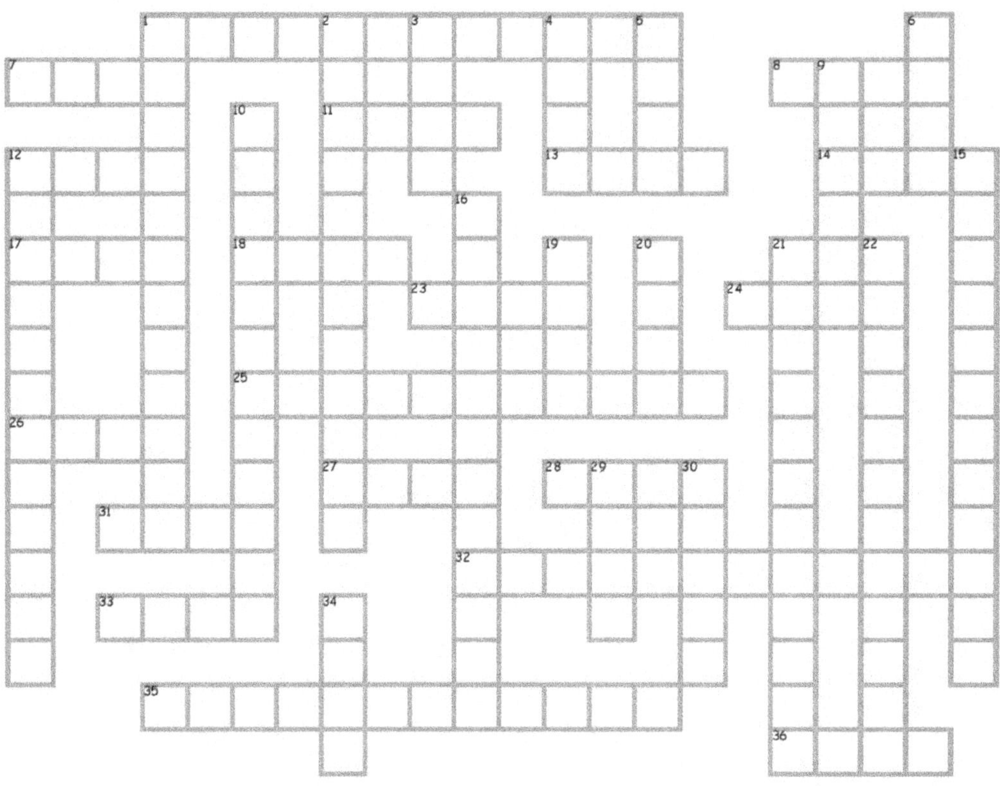

Across

1 following a meal
7 r- breathe
8 s-study of
11 r- eye
12 pert to -s
13 Methicillin Resistant Stapholococus Aureus- extremely virulent staph infection, can be fatal; use contact isolation - gloves and gown
14 middle coat of eyeball, includes iris, ciliary body, choroid
17 r- to lead
18 mass of fibrin and cells that is prod in a wound
23 r- destroy
24 physical evidence of a disease process
25 recanalization of blood vessel by surgery
26 r- gland
27 sebum -r
28 r- sight
31 r- breast
32 laparoscopic ____
33 colored portion of eye w/pupil in center
35 laparoscopic ____
36 r/cf -thread

Down

1 deficiency of ALL types of blood cells **
2 surg spe in disease of anus and rectum
3 terminal end of digestivve tract *
4 insuline dependent diabetes mellitus; type 1 diabetes,
5 transparent refractive struc behind iris
6 r- cell
9 condition -s
10 inflammation of pancreas, causes difficulty regulating insulin and sugar
12 pert to being inside the trachea
15 white blood cell w/o granules in cytoplasm
16 w/o symptoms or abnormalities
19 beyond, subsequent to -p
20 r- mind
21 pouchlike opening or sac from tubualr structure (eg intestine)
22 specialist for intestines
29 r- paralysis
30 male
34 r- spinal cord

Nursing Medical Terminology

Matching Worksheets

Med Terminol Matching

Write the code corresponding to the correct match in the space provided.

___ 1. catabolism

___ 2. al

___ 3. par

___ 4. pustule

___ 5. patell

___ 6. nervous system

___ 7. blast

___ 8. otoscope

___ 9. autologous blood donation

___ 10. sacr

___ 11. neur/o

___ 12. carbuncle

___ 13. intussusception

___ 14. sin/o

___ 15. vol

___ 16. lip/o

___ 17. metastasis

___ 18. dors

___ 19. stoma

___ 20. tibia

___ 21. plate

___ 22. anastom

___ 23. de

___ 24. intus

___ 25. anus

___ 26. necr/o

___ 27. functions of skeletal muscle

___ 28. CPAP

___ 29. morph

___ 30. angi/o

___ 31. ster

___ 32. AHD

___ 33. dementia

___ 34. VEP

___ 35. ASD

___ 36. ism

___ 37. bi

___ 38. open (comminuted)

A1. p- removal, without

B1. transfusion w/ own blood

C1. fluid, noncellular part of blood

D1. around -p

E1. immune rxn directed against a person's own tissues

F1. not -p

G1. surg remov of plaque from artery

H1. r-stone

I1. blood sugar, breath sounds, bowel sounds

J1. tube linking pharynx and stomach

K1. incise, cut -r

L1. incomplete bony ring that attaches the upper limb to the axial skeleton **

M1. formation -s

N1. physical evidence of a disease process

O1. gland

P1. shortness of breath

Q1. pertaining to mucus or the mucosa

R1. throb-r

S1. r- gray matter

T1. state of muscular contraction *

U1. bent, humpback-r

V1. skin

W1. itching

X1. inflammation of gums*

Y1. chronic dilation of bronchi following inflamm disease and obstruction

Z1. surg proc to change the size or shape of the nose

A2. poisonous subst form by cell or organism

B2. upper respiratory infection

C2. protein of muscle that stores and transports O2

D2. p- two

E2. under (behind) the sternum

F2. structure -s

G2. * inability to coordinate muscle activity leading to jerky movements

H2. eczema -r/cf

I2. r- digest

J2. hormone that promotes masculine characteristics

fracture

___ 39. proct

___ 40. ex

___ 41. pathy

___ 42. Crohn disease

___ 43. violet

___ 44. nutrient

___ 45. ad

___ 46. umbilical

___ 47. arthrodesis

___ 48. cervical

___ 49. anterior

___ 50. ory

___ 51. collateral

___ 52. ectomy

___ 53. pleurisy

___ 54. pancreatitis

___ 55. a

___ 56. louse lice (pl)

___ 57. ism

___ 58. zygoma

___ 59. 4 primary tissue groups

___ 60. glaucoma

___ 61. in

___ 62. tamponade

___ 63. masticate

___ 64. strain

___ 65. contract

___ 66. de

___ 67. insulin

___ 68. posterior

___ 69. hypertension

___ 70. con

___ 71. ossicle

___ 72. aneurysm

___ 73. hiat

___ 74. otitis media

___ 75. hernia

___ 76. complete fracture

___ 77. a

___ 78. perforat

___ 79. graine

___ 80. stasis

K2. 1 of 3 muscles in buttocks

L2. area of dead tissue-r

M2. contraction-r

N2. any small projection

O2. inflamm of gray matter of spinal cord, leading to paralsis of limbs and muscles of Respiration

P2. lymphatic vessels-r

Q2. to form-r

R2. clear, gelatinous substance that forms the substance of a cell, except for the nucleus

S2. pert to belly or situated nearer to surface of body

T2. reduction in diameter of a blood vessel

U2. membrane that lines the interior of freely moving joints

V2. to puncture

W2. failure or incomplete dev of pathways of visionto brain; lazy eye *

X2. s- condition,process

Y2. hardness-r

Z2. sleep-r

A3. place -r

B3. defense mech from antibodies in blood

C3. formation -s

D3. thin wall separting 2 cavities or 2 tissue masses; (latin) a partition

E3. to without a blood supply

F3. r - granule, cartilage

G3. change-s

H3. sheet of fibrous connective tissue; latin - a band **

I3. cond in which bones become more porous, brittle, and fragile, more likely to fracture; from loss of bone density

J3. together, union, association, - p

K3. roof of mouth, floor of nose

L3. s- pertaining to

M3. bone that forms part of the base and sides of the skull

N3. r- eardrum

O3. their granuales take up purple stain equally, whterh acid or alkaline

P3. skull

Q3. bones, cartilage, tendons, ligaments

R3. take away-p

S3. action, condition -s

T3. r - efficient, practical

U3. r- frenzy

V3. small head -r

W3. pertaining to -s

___ 81. greenstick fx

___ 82. pancytopenia

___ 83. neo

___ 84. plasm

___ 85. pancreat

___ 86. perforat

___ 87. phalanx, phalanges (pl)

___ 88. connective tissue

___ 89. retrovirus

___ 90. pharnyx

___ 91. melanin

___ 92. MRSA

___ 93. encephal

___ 94. flex

___ 95. membran

___ 96. umbilic

___ 97. thrombus

___ 98. epicardium

___ 99. apnea

___ 100. trachea

___ 101. sarc

___ 102. duodenal

___ 103. diastole

___ 104. mitochondria

___ 105. pectoral

___ 106. capsule

___ 107. terat

___ 108. biceps brachii

___ 109. croup

___ 110. spin

___ 111. pepsin

___ 112. oma

___ 113. dis

___ 114. excis

___ 115. poplit/e

___ 116. pm

___ 117. cerebrum

___ 118. synovial membrane

___ 119. ent

___ 120. medulla

___ 121. systole

___ 122. ACL

___ 123. PNB

X3. pertaining to the back surface of the body, situated behind

Y3. r- poison

Z3. connective, epithelial, muscle, nervous

A4. two -p

B4. normal breathing, 12-20 / min

C4. in front of the patella

D4. fibrous band that connects muscle to bone

E4. arteriosclerotic heart disease

F4. many-p

G4. r-ear

H4. parasitic insect

I4. below normal level of oxygen in tissues, gases, or blood

J4. r-press together

K4. s- pertaining to

L4. surgical removal of gallbladder by laparoscope/endoscope

M4. pertaining to the heart and blood vessels

N4. yellow staining of tissues w/bile pigments, including bilirubin

O4. surg removal of adipose tissue using suction

P4. bone is broken, but skin is not broken

Q4. pathologic death of cells or tissue **

R4. patella -r

S4. backward flow; (latin)backward flow

T4. test for decubitus ulcer- touch reddened area and it does not turn white- if stays red - sign of stage 1 skin break down

U4. pert to digestive tract

V4. latin-stand out

W4. excessive prod of thryroid hormone; increases body metabolism, including protruding eyes, tachycardia, htn, diaphoresis, treamor, anxiety, diarrhea, weight loss

X4. disease of heart muscle, the myocardium

Y4. r-twelve

Z4. r-mouth

A5. shape-r

B5. abnormal increas of CO2 in arterial bloodstream

C5. inflammation of gallbladder

D5. shoulder blade

E5. dilated, tortuous vein

F5. r - before

G5. Methicillin Resistant Stapholococus Aureus- extremely virulent staph infection, can be fatal; use contact isolation - gloves and gown

H5. skin eruption

I5. p- small

___ 124. ize	J5. foreign -p
___ 125. uvula	K5. unknown-r
___ 126. cyst	L5. small mass within the nucleus
___ 127. ior	M5. s- pertaining to
___ 128. gastr	N5. immune rxn directed against person's own tissue
___ 129. hyper	O5. r- bladder
___ 130. abdomin/o	P5. r/cf - nucleus
___ 131. pector	Q5. s- pertaining to
___ 132. SQ	R5. bone of tarsus (foot) that forms the heel
___ 133. migraine	S5. single bone of upper arm; latin-shoulder
___ 134. thromboembolism	T5. protrusion of eyeball
___ 135. lobe	U5. surgical excision -s
___ 136. sympathetic nervous system	V5. artificial part to remedy defect in body; greek - addition
___ 137. lact	W5. excessive ketones in blood making it acid
___ 138. ultra	X5. fx is at right angles to the long axis of the bone
___ 139. cardiomyopathy	Y5. cancer
___ 140. pnea	Z5. electrocardiogram
___ 141. staphylococcus aurus	A6. inflamm of small bronchioles
___ 142. pulmonary	B6. r- kidney
___ 143. epi	C6. weaken the ability of organism to prod disease
___ 144. acromion	D6. pertaining to the lungs
___ 145. atrophy	E6. large intestine, expanding from cecum to rectum *
___ 146. skull - number of bones	F6. waves of alternate contraction and relaxation of intest wall to move food along diges tract *
___ 147. adrenal gland	G6. r- esophagus
___ 148. hyperpnea	H6. having 3 parts; tricuspid heart valve has 3 flaps
___ 149. itis	I6. chemical formed in one tissue or organ and carried by the blood to stimulate or inhibit a function of another tissue or organ; (Greek) set in motion
___ 150. carpal tunnel syndrome CNS)	J6. pain in various parts of the musculoskeletal sys
___ 151. dys	K6. auricle - external ear
___ 152. mitral	L6. substance that reduces or relieves the response to pain w/o prod loss of consciousness
___ 153. cholelithiasis	M6. a bone-forming cell
___ 154. IDDM	N6. any small projection
___ 155. or/o	O6. low oxygen level in arterial blood
___ 156. AED	P6. per to disease attacking the population of very large area
___ 157. mit/o	Q6. constriction, stenosis, particularly of aorta
___ 158. epi	R6. lower end of femur, flat end of tibia, patella, fibula
___ 159. tx	S6. skin
___ 160. vasoconstriction	T6. r- constrict
___ 161. fusion	U6. ventricular tachycardia- rapid heart beat occuring in ventricles
___ 162. embolus	V6. right sided heart failure arising from chronic lung disease
___ 163. skelet	W6. death -r
___ 164. brachi/i	
___ 165. home/o	

___ 166. complement	X6. without --p
___ 167. gastrin	Y6. s - conditionn
___ 168. prosthesis	Z6. inflammation of a bursa
___ 169. hypo	A7. front surface of the body;
___ 170. Ab	B7. r- pressure
___ 171. pallor	C7. fibrous band that connects muscle to bone
___ 172. myel	D7. neck -r
___ 173. ease	E7. nose -r
___ 174. supine	F7. parotid gland is salivary gland beside ear
___ 175. cirrh	G7. ventricular fibrillation -occurs when ventricles lose control, quivering instead of pumping
___ 176. de	H7. band of fibrous tissue connectin 2 structures; latin - band, sheet
___ 177. meta	I7. p- from, out of, removal, out of
___ 178. calcaneal tendon	J7. s- take action
___ 179. petit mal	K7. the body as a whole -r
___ 180. ing	L7. substance that, when dissolved in a suitable medium, forms electrically charged particles
___ 181. mandible	M7. lyint face up, flat on spine
___ 182. SX	N7. mass of fibrin and cells that is prod in a wound
___ 183. tongue	O7. maintaining the stability of a system or the body's internal environment
___ 184. ileum	P7. hole thru wall of a structure
___ 185. abrasion	Q7. turning eye inward toward nose; cross-eyed
___ 186. fract	R7. r - bone
___ 187. intradermal	S7. bone-r
___ 188. clavicle	T7. disease -s
___ 189. CA	U7. calcaneus -r
___ 190. respiration	V7. back-r
___ 191. ly	W7. endocrine gland o upper pole of each kikney
___ 192. logist	X7. inflammatino of stomach and intestines; stomach flu *
___ 193. megaly	Y7. s- disease
___ 194. ation	Z7. from inflamm and swelling of overused tendon sheaths; repetitive movements can cause it
___ 195. interstitial	A8. skeleton -
___ 196. hist/o	B8. r- armpit
___ 197. hypertrophy	C8. polymorphonuclear leukocyte
___ 198. ASHD	D8. waves of alternate contraction and relaxation of intestinal wall to move food along digestive tract: feeling you have to have BM *
___ 199. epiphysis	E8. chronic, progressive, irreversible loss of mind's cognitive and intellectual functions
___ 200. genesis	F8. infection of the scalp - ringworm
___ 201. peri	G8. small red blood cell
___ 202. phagocytose	H8. pert to tarsus
___ 203. C/O	
___ 204. cori	
___ 205. pnea	
___ 206. psychosis	
___ 207. bipolar disorder	
___ 208. pneumon	

___ 209. cyanosis

___ 210. arthr/o

___ 211. or

___ 212. pronat

___ 213. septum septa (pl)

___ 214. myel

___ 215. syndrome

___ 216. dermat/o

___ 217. fibr/o

___ 218. some

___ 219. bilirubin

___ 220. metabolic acidosis

___ 221. dermis

___ 222. gastroenterologist

___ 223. osteocyte

___ 224. dorsi

___ 225. mal

___ 226. ketoacidosis

___ 227. connective tissue

___ 228. osis

___ 229. ostomy

___ 230. A+O

___ 231. anastomosis

___ 232. perinatal

___ 233. aorta

___ 234. prone

___ 235. pectoral girdle

___ 236. SOB

___ 237. lash

___ 238. alignment

___ 239. h+P

___ 240. exudate

___ 241. necr/o

___ 242. let

___ 243. orex

___ 244. AC

___ 245. organ

___ 246. cubitus

___ 247. esotropia

___ 248. cirrh

___ 249. patella, pattellae (pl)

___ 250. scoliosis

___ 251. duct

I8. pubis -r

J8. p- around

K8. r- knowledge

L8. muscle of arm that has 3 heads or points of origin **

M8. makes absorption of vit B12 happen

N8. r - hollow space

O8. horizontal plane div body into uper and lower portions (superior and inferior)

P8. occurs when interference in cardiac electrical conduction prevents atria's contraction from coordinating w/ventricles' contractions

Q8. genetic disorder among Afro Amer. RBCs form in sickle shape

R8. metabolic syndrome caused by absolute or relative insulin deficiency and/or ineffectiveness

S8. s - pertaining to

T8. cond - bone marrow unable to prod suffic red cells, white cells, and platelets

U8. dark blue -r

V8. graft from another species (not human)

W8. internal invasion, infection -r

X8. shaped like mitre (bishop wears); mitral valve-

Y8. mandible -r

Z8. chronic anemia due to lack of vit B12 **

A9. neurotransmitter in some specific small areas of the brain

B9. r-breath

C9. pertaining to

D9. smooth articular surf of bone on which another glides

E9. capable of being transmitted; a disease caused by the action of a microorganism

F9. air in the pleural cavity

G9. mouth of windpipe-r

H9. myocardial infarct - heart attack

I9. diagnosis

J9. area between lungs containing the heart, aorta, venae cavae, esophagus

K9. p - in

L9. atrial septal defect

M9. puncture -s

N9. pouchlike opening or sac from tubualr structure (eg intestine)

O9. upset stomach, epigastric pain, nausea, gas

P9. r- bore through

Q9. presence of gallstone in common bile duct

R9. p- half, derivied from hemi

S9. the same - r

_____ 252. cell

_____ 253. gastroesophageal

_____ 254. laparoscopic
     cholesectomy

_____ 255. suscept

_____ 256. coccyx

_____ 257. blepharoplasty

_____ 258. melanin

_____ 259. thesis

_____ 260. insulin

_____ 261. nucle/o

_____ 262. orth/o

_____ 263. intrins

_____ 264. peri

_____ 265. lacrimal

_____ 266. glut

_____ 267. CXR

_____ 268. polyuria

_____ 269. globin

_____ 270. subcutaneus

_____ 271. ale

_____ 272. pneumo

_____ 273. pinna

_____ 274. coronal

_____ 275. presbyopia

_____ 276. P

_____ 277. Tourette syndrome

_____ 278. ismus

_____ 279. anastomosis

_____ 280. conception

_____ 281. thymus

_____ 282. toxin

_____ 283. oid

_____ 284. non

_____ 285. iatry

_____ 286. skelet

_____ 287. SOB

_____ 288. peptic

_____ 289. paraplegia

_____ 290. por/o

_____ 291. dysphagia

_____ 292. meniscectomy

_____ 293. aspiration

_____ 294. stax

T9. coronary heart disease

U9. treatment-r

V9. fluid-r

W9. semifluid, partially digested food passed from stomach
into duodenum

X9. lack of blood supply to a tissue

Y9. organ surrounding the urethra at base of male urinary
bladder; (Greek) one who stands before

Z9. belly-r

A10. fleshy projection of the soft palate

B10. one -r

C10. before the time of birth

D10. decreased no of red blood cells

E10. blind pouch that is 1st part of large intestine

F10. bad, difficult -p

G10. s- inflammation

H10. aphthous ulcer, erosion of mucous membrane lining the
mouth *

I10. 3rd portion of small intestine

J10. running-r

K10. liquid containing suspended particles

L10. stretching or enlarging an opening or structure

M10. r- sensation of pain

N10. pert to correction and cure of deformities and diseases of
musculoskeletal sys

O10. in front of the elbow **

P10. complete or partial opacity of lens

Q10. r/cf -thread

R10. burn from contact with hot water or steam

S10. agent capable of dissolving or liquefying mucus

T10. r- arrow

U10. med spec in disease of ear

V10. skin -r

W10. cell

X10. substance that causes clotting

Y10. s- tissue

Z10. r/cf - ketone

A11. chronic anemia due to lack of Vit B12

B11. chronic inflammatory disease of joints

C11. per to disease always present in a community

D11. collection of blood that escaped from vessels into
surrounding tissue

E11. space at entrance to canal

F11. abnormal condition

____ 295. Hodgkin

____ 296. myopia

____ 297. viscosity

____ 298. SARS

____ 299. bile

____ 300. hypercapnia

____ 301. erythemat

____ 302. tinea cruris

____ 303. bilateral

____ 304. regenerate

____ 305. blephar/o

____ 306. pneumothorax

____ 307. cutaneus

____ 308. ili

____ 309. UTI

____ 310. ot

____ 311. palat

____ 312. ven

____ 313. dentine

____ 314. rotator cuff

____ 315. bi

____ 316. rhin

____ 317. arthroscopy

____ 318. arthrodesis

____ 319. palpit

____ 320. CDiff

____ 321. hyperthyroidism

____ 322. scapula

____ 323. algia

____ 324. infectious

____ 325. tachypnea

____ 326. ischi

____ 327. bariatric

____ 328. therapeut

____ 329. thorax

____ 330. Ab

____ 331. cartilage

____ 332. multidisciplinary

____ 333. penia

____ 334. comminut

____ 335. autoimmune

____ 336. aden

____ 337. plasia

G11. proc or dx with name derived from name of person who discovered it

H11. clavicle -r

I11. r- gums

J11. spherical mass of cells containing a cavity, eg. hair follicle

K11. s - small

L11. pus in a body cavity, particularly in pleural cavity

M11. r- within

N11. deficient number of WBCs

O11. self gov visceral motor div of peripheral nerv sys

P11. upper jaw bone, containing rt and lt maxillary sinuses;

Q11. surgical removal of gallbladder (cyst-gb)

R11. community aquired MRSA- methicillin resistant staphylococcus aureus

S11. strange, other -r

T11. r- nose

U11. acute clinical event caused by impaired cerebral circulation

V11. radius -r

W11. mass of lymph tiss on either side of throat @ back of tongue

X11. blood vessel-r

Y11. canal leading from bladder to the outside

Z11. stone

A12. pain in muscle fibers **

B12. r/cf - cell

C12. together, with -p

D12. most-s

E12. without -p

F12. anterior cruciate ligament - at front of knee,

G12. nature-r

H12. hives, small, itchy swelling of the skin; However, wheals raised by an injection do not itch

I12. antibody -protein prod in response to an antigen

J12. removal of specific part of organ or structure

K12. excessive eating

L12. with the muscle

M12. fascia (skin)

N12. thrush; the most common form of candida; can prod recurrent infections of the skin, nails, and mucous membranes

O12. pertaining to birth

P12. kneecap; thin, circular bone in front of knee joint, embedded in the patellar tendon; laint - small plate

Q12. with

___ 338. PVC	R12. increase in size, but not in number, of an indiv tissue element **
___ 339. endocrine	S12. r - patella
___ 340. humoral immunity	T12. connective tissue layer of the skin beneath the epidermis; middle of 3 layers of skin
___ 341. otolith	U12. gland-r
___ 342. classification of bones	V12. femur -r
___ 343. tampon	W12. body's largest organ,in RUQ abdomen
___ 344. lith	X12. cut into
___ 345. dx	Y12. a joint
___ 346. colostomy	Z12. press together, narrow-r
___ 347. endocardium	A13. postural drainage therapy
___ 348. supinat	B13. slipping of 1 part of bowel inside another to cause obstruction
___ 349. radius	C13. back of the skull
___ 350. infection	D13. r- nose
___ 351. dyspepsia	E13. smallest unit of the body capable of independent existence; (latin) storeroom
___ 352. dyspnea	F13. enlargement of the heart
___ 353. hypothalamus	G13. fluid filled cyst, or collection of nerve cells outside the brain and spinal cord
___ 354. ity	H13. opening thru a structure
___ 355. nutri	I13. mucous membrane
___ 356. coron	J13. high density lipoprotein - good cholesterol
___ 357. astigmatism	K13. part of capsule of the shoulder joint **
___ 358. intravenous	L13. slow breathing, less than 10/min
___ 359. coarctation	M13. med spec of disease of the heart
___ 360. basophil	N13. cond - spleen removes blood components at excessive rate **
___ 361. fascia	O13. shell- like external ear
___ 362. atrium	P13. insulent dependent diabetes mellitus
___ 363. paranoia	Q13. acquired w/i a hospital
___ 364. epilept	R13. functional center of a cell or structure; (latin) command center
___ 365. syn	S13. collection of similar cells; (latin)- to weave
___ 366. gen	T13. an incomplete dislocation when some contact between the joint surfaces remains
___ 367. cortic	U13. protein formed by liver; converted to thrombin in blood clotting mechanism
___ 368. incomplete freacture	V13. increase in diameter of a blood vessel
___ 369. periosteum	W13. hair loss, baldness
___ 370. atelectasis	X13. wedge-shaped bone at the base of the skull
___ 371. scler	Y13. hard protein -r
___ 372. hypoglycemia	Z13. inflamm of middle ear
___ 373. anemia	A14. having a structure in its corerct postion relative to others
___ 374. tendin	B14. r - rectum
___ 375. capn (r)	
___ 376. ate	
___ 377. al, ic, ory	
___ 378. nonblanchable erythema	
___ 379. cardiovascular	
___ 380. ure	

___ 381. thromb/o

___ 382. grand mal seizure

___ 383. humor

___ 384. pectoral

___ 385. plas

___ 386. gen

___ 387. sect (r)

___ 388. herpes zoster

___ 389. version

___ 390. occipit

___ 391. candida albicans

___ 392. leukemia

___ 393. tempor

___ 394. arthroscopy

___ 395. dis

___ 396. allograft

___ 397. dermat

___ 398. neutrophil

___ 399. hetero

___ 400. cortex

___ 401. maxilla

___ 402. scleroderma

___ 403. lipectomy

___ 404. parasit

___ 405. oma

___ 406. glyc

___ 407. pre

___ 408. atel (r)

___ 409. 5 regions of vertebral column

___ 410. digestion

___ 411. emuls

___ 412. tomy

___ 413. laryngopharynx

___ 414. delt

___ 415. rhabdomyolysis

___ 416. carcin

___ 417. derm

___ 418. whip

___ 419. idiopathic

___ 420. excrete

___ 421. peripheral vision

___ 422. phagia

___ 423. articulate

C14. ear was

D14. exit area of stomach

E14. pertaining to

F14. r/cf - heart

G14. blood vessel -r

H14. r - to make fruitful

I14. on side of knee, located outside the knee joint; most common ligament damaged in sports injuries

J14. cut or surgical wound

K14. r- brain

L14. r- focus

M14. through-p

N14. p- within, inside

O14. breathe -r

P14. r- hernia

Q14. process of using an instrument to examine visually

R14. surg proc to chang the size or shape of the breast

S14. lower part of the uterus

T14. s - to examine, to view

U14. r - back

V14. r- malformed fetus, monster

W14. med specialty of stomach and intestines *

X14. anteroposterior

Y14. r-abdomen in general

Z14. r- treatment

A15. revive from apparent death -r **

B15. inherited cond when bone formation is incomplete, leading to fragile, easily broken bones

C15. fibrous tissue layer surrounding a joint or other structure; (latin) little box

D15. * inflammation of meninges, bacterial or viral; vaccination available !

E15. s - process, condition

F15. 8 carpal bones of wrist

G15. prod internal or hormonal secretion

H15. myocardial infarct - heart attack

I15. old English-band-r

J15. r - chest

K15. waxy secretion of the sebaceous glands

L15. toward-p

M15. below the skin; same as hypodermic; 3rd layer of skin, deepest

N15. within the epidermis (top layer of skin)

O15. pertaining to the back or situated behind

___ 424. strict

___ 425. varic

___ 426. photoreceptor

___ 427. debridement

___ 428. urethra

___ 429. pancreas

___ 430. OA

___ 431. tissue

___ 432. laryngotracheobronchitis

___ 433. laryng

___ 434. sarcoidosis

___ 435. cyan (r)

___ 436. capillary

___ 437. parasite

___ 438. sebum

___ 439. hemolysis

___ 440. erythroblastosis fetalis

___ 441. keratin

___ 442. autograft

___ 443. islets of Langerhans

___ 444. VSD

___ 445. aplastic anemia

___ 446. prand

___ 447. congest

___ 448. ceps

___ 449. eczem/a

___ 450. phylac

___ 451. cornea

___ 452. pariet

___ 453. anabol

___ 454. fibromyalgia

___ 455. proct

___ 456. synov

___ 457. menisc

___ 458. pancreas

___ 459. intrinsic factor

___ 460. canker sore

___ 461. ulcer

___ 462. cirrhosis

___ 463. cellul

___ 464. nos/o

___ 465. amin

___ 466. neuropathy

P15. between atria of the heart

Q15. r/cf - joint

R15. armpit

S15. of the arm -r

T15. pertaining to one side of the body

U15. 5 parallel bones of the foot between the tarsus and phalanges

V15. same, alike -p

W15. vertebra -r

X15. disease -r

Y15. carries blood from intestines to liver

Z15. having the funtion of

A16. wrench or tear in ligament

B16. inflammation of tendon

C16. gluteus maximus muscle is larges muscle in body, covering large part of each buttock **

D16. stick together to form clumps **

E16. tension present in resting muscles

F16. s- pertaining to

G16. after, subsequent to -p

H16. * degenerative disease of retina

I16. removal, out of -p

J16. sweat-r

K16. breastbone

L16. s- pertaining to

M16. r- breast

N16. muscle - r

O16. large wing shaped bone at the upper and posterior part of pelvis

P16. tissue consisting of contractile cells

Q16. congenital lesion of the skin; (latin) mole, birthmark

R16. lead-r

S16. acute myocardial infarction - heart attack

T16. beyond, subsequent to -p

U16. double layer of membranes surrounding the heart **

V16. segement of small intestine between duodenum and ileum

W16. s - small

X16. aspiration of fluid from a joint

Y16. feel good hormone; neurotransmitter in CNS and PNS

Z16. modd disorder with alternating periods of depression and mania

A17. detailed skin assessment tool

B17. r- tympanic membrane

C17. contraction of the heart muscle

___ 467. orthot	D17. structure
___ 468. - s	E17. suffering from low bp (hypotension)
___ 469. auricle	F17. hypertension
___ 470. origin	G17. surgical incision
___ 471. verruca	H17. r- breathe
___ 472. enterologist	I17. r/cf - tissue
___ 473. ileostomy	J17. pertaining to one side of the body
___ 474. anatomy	K17. med specialty concerned w/disorders of the skin
___ 475. prenatal	L17. break into pieces -r
___ 476. cyt/o	M17. mandible -r
___ 477. um	N17. below -p
___ 478. photophobia	O17. terminal part of colon from sigmoid to anal canal (inside) *
___ 479. pandemic	
___ 480. platelet	P17. to break -r
___ 481. ur/o	Q17. diseasese
___ 482. impetigo	R17. r-throat
___ 483. lipase	S17. passage thru skin, as by needle puncture
___ 484. occult blood	T17. s- abnormal condition
___ 485. meta	U17. r-bitter
___ 486. ischium, ischia (pl)	V17. milky fluid that results from digestion and absorption of fats in small intestine
___ 487. immune	W17. 3 layered covering of the brain and spinal cord *
___ 488. gastric	X17. fluid secreted by liver into duodenum
___ 489. epilepsy	Y17. hole thu wall of a structure
___ 490. tibi	Z17. muscle that helps flex forearm **
___ 491. tympan	A18. delicate inner layer of meninges
___ 492. ketoacidosis	B18. injujry to brain at point directly opposite point of contact
___ 493. volunt	C18. spread of a disease from one part of the body to another
___ 494. vas/o	D18. treatment
___ 495. carcinoma	E18. r- stretch over
___ 496. all	F18. excessive thirst
___ 497. alopecia	G18. bone is pulled from distal end back into algnment through a proc called reduction, often under anesthesia
___ 498. mandibul	H18. urine
___ 499. cellulitis	I18. r- ear
___ 500. CAO	J18. simoid colon is shaped like "s"
___ 501. meningitis	K18. r- to fight
___ 502. ot	L18. r- sugar, glycogen
___ 503. centesis	M18. single mass of a substance, Greek-lump
___ 504. meniscus	N18. r- beyond
___ 505. toxi	O18. a tissue consisting of cells that can contract
___ 506. cholecystitis	P18. r-island
___ 507. capsul	Q18. decreased calcification of bone, low bone density
___ 508. lysis	R18. destroy-r
___ 509. tic	

____ 510. uvula

____ 511. protocol

____ 512. TIA

____ 513. nephr

____ 514. esophag

____ 515. cerumen

____ 516. ten/o

____ 517. stoma

____ 518. derm

____ 519. tom

____ 520. adenoid

____ 521. NKA

____ 522. malign

____ 523. rosacea

____ 524. exotropia

____ 525. bride

____ 526. intestine

____ 527. hale (r)

____ 528. colostomy

____ 529. later

____ 530. scabies

____ 531. implantable

____ 532. androgen

____ 533. media

____ 534. hyper

____ 535. hypersplenism

____ 536. liposuction

____ 537. vascul

____ 538. retinopathy

____ 539. peps

____ 540. atory

____ 541. mucolytic

____ 542. atrioventricular (AV)

____ 543. pericardium

____ 544. constrict

____ 545. crine

____ 546. suscept

____ 547. synovial fluid

____ 548. artery

____ 549. dysentery

____ 550. varices (sing-varix)

____ 551. melatonin

____ 552. rotat

S18. disease in whihc the body makes antibodies directed against its own tissues; fights self

T18. skin hemorrhages, initially red, then turn purple

U18. trans ischemic attack - mini stroke

V18. resistance of fluid to flow

W18. bone that forms the prominence of the cheek

X18. a swelling at the base of the big toe

Y18. looking inside

Z18. p- after

A19. complains of

B19. inflamm of lining of rectum

C19. without appetite

D19. 3rd portion of small intestine

E19. lining of a tubular structure that secretes

F19. process -s

G19. life-r

H19. r-fat

I19. r- abdomen

J19. large wing-shaped bone at the upper and posterior part of the pelvis (Latin) groin

K19. r-digestion

L19. pertaining to

M19. r- eardrum

N19. light sensitive innermost layer of eyeball

O19. formation-r

P19. joint -r

Q19. pertaining to

R19. semifluid, partially digested food passed from stomach into duodenum

S19. pertaining to the macrocyte (large red blood cell)

T19. by shape: long, short - (wrist, ankle, patella) ,flat- (skull,ribs), irregular(vertebrae)

U19. treatment

V19. r-enzyme, fermenting

W19. inflamm of conjunctiva- inner lining of eyelids

X19. maxilla -r

Y19. excessive production of urine

Z19. hard

A20. protect-r

B20. middle coat of eyeball, includes iris, ciliary body, choroid

C20. extremely high body temperature or fever

D20. skin disease prod by mites; (latin) to scratch

E20. to close, plug, or completely obstruct

F20. lymph tissue in midline at back of throat*

___ 553. symptomat

___ 554. sign

___ 555. tropin

___ 556. MI

___ 557. anthrac (r)

___ 558. cuff

___ 559. al

___ 560. visual acuity

___ 561. natal

___ 562. thrush

___ 563. AC

___ 564. otorhinolaryngologist

___ 565. triceps brachii

___ 566. calvicul

___ 567. colloid

___ 568. s/p

___ 569. UTI

___ 570. melena

___ 571. ole

___ 572. chrom/o

___ 573. tinea pedis

___ 574. diaphoresis

___ 575. anxiety

___ 576. chronic

___ 577. polyp

___ 578. kerat

___ 579. biopsy

___ 580. resuscit

___ 581. hormon

___ 582. interventricular (IV)

___ 583. HTN

___ 584. epigastric

___ 585. ethm

___ 586. drome

___ 587. epistaxis

___ 588. Braden Risk Assessment scale

___ 589. tracheotomy

___ 590. postprandial

___ 591. mucus

___ 592. Kaposi sarcoma

___ 593. BS

___ 594. macule

___ 595. glottis or glott

G20. r- appetite

H20. removal by suction of fluid or gas from a body cavity

I20. inflammation of fascia prod deat of the tissue

J20. * mild brain injury; brain bruise

K20. x-ray of a joint taken after injection of a contrast medium into the joint

L20. terminal end of digestivve tract *

M20. mood disorder w/hperactivity, irritability, and rapid speech

N20. its granules attract a rosy-red color on staining

O20. s-study of

P20. nothing by mouth

Q20. pulling or dragging force, latin - to pull

R20. tear or jagged wound of the skin caused by blunt trauma; not a cut

S20. fx of distal radius at wrist

T20. artery-r

U20. result of -s

V20. difficulty swallowing

W20. itch

X20. departure from normal health exper by patient

Y20. chamber of heart - pumps blood; also means a cavity in the brain (prod cerebrospinal fluid) **

Z20. infection aquired while in the hospital

A21. main trunk of systemic arterial sys

B21. s- new opening

C21. r-twelve

D21. r - tail

E21. general term for a group of realted skin infections caused by different species of fungi; (latin) worm

F21. wart casued by a virus (latin) wart

G21. self -p

H21. a flow -

I21. r- birth, born

J21. of the back -r

K21. muscle of arm that has 2 heads or points of origin on scapula **

L21. turning eye outward away from nose

M21. small, circumscribed elevation of the skin; (latin) pimple

N21. destruction of muscle to prod myoglobin

O21. s- pertaining to, quality of

P21. substance that surrounds and protects cells, is maufactured by the cells, and holds them together; (latin) mater-mother

Q21. forecast of the probable future course and outcome of a disease

___ 596. HAV, HBV, HCV

___ 597. bursa

___ 598. muscle

___ 599. systemic lupus

___ 600. tars

___ 601. tens

___ 602. rash

___ 603. nephr

___ 604. antigen

___ 605. adipose

___ 606. ultraviolet

___ 607. pathy

___ 608. angiography

___ 609. tallus

___ 610. SRD

___ 611. plasm

___ 612. valgus

___ 613. lumbar

___ 614. zygomat

___ 615. spine

___ 616. endoscopy

___ 617. palatine

___ 618. jaundice

___ 619. ant

___ 620. arteri/o

___ 621. cusp

___ 622. plasty

___ 623. ather

___ 624. medi

___ 625. lith

___ 626. PMNL

___ 627. amin(e)

___ 628. scler/o

___ 629. pia mater

___ 630. cytoplasm

___ 631. mediastinum

___ 632. cholecystectomy

___ 633. vertebr

___ 634. plasty

___ 635. micro

___ 636. hypothalamus

___ 637. uni

___ 638. proctitis

R21. fx consists of 1 bone fragment driven into another, resulting in shortening of the limb

S21. blood clot-r

T21. skin graft from another person or cadaver; (same as allograft)

U21. by mouth

V21. inflamm of pleura - membrane covering lungs and lining ribs in thoracic cavity

W21. in-p

X21. hormone that mobilizes glucose from body storage

Y21. lying down -r

Z21. band of muscle that encircles an opening: when it contracts, the opening squeezes closed *

A22. fatty, blood-forming tissue in the cavities of long bones

B22. major protein of connective tissue, cartilage, and bone

C22. thin, hairlike projection, particularly of mucous membrane lining a cavity

D22. burnt, dead tissue lying on top of 3rd degree burns;

E22. r- narrow

F22. complex of cell and chemical reactions occurring in response to an injury or chemical or biologic agent

G22. arm-r

H22. r- white of eye, hardness *

I22. backward -p

J22. result when extra impulses arise from a ventricle, 2. v-fib- ventricular fibrillation -occurs when ventricles lose control, quivering instead of pumping

K22. lying face down on belly

L22. a fragment of the fractured bone breaks the skin, or a wound extends to the site of the fx

M22. muscle

N22. the study of the causes of a disease

O22. enlargement-s

P22. body's prin carb reserve, stored in liver and skeletal muscle

Q22. brain, spinal cord, nerves, and sensory receptors, funct: rapidly coordinates body functions and enables learning and memory

R22. tendon -r

S22. pert to stomach and esophagus

T22. the people-r

U22. r - cover, skin

V22. nearer to the middle of the body

W22. tube from back of nose to larnyx (back of throat)

X22. strand or filament; latin -fiber

Y22. s- state, condition

___ 639. sis

___ 640. pepsinogen

___ 641. DVT

___ 642. bronchiectasis

___ 643. cutan/e

___ 644. connect

___ 645. CAD

___ 646. emuls

___ 647. Heberden node

___ 648. idiopathic

___ 649. lingu

___ 650. clavicul

___ 651. plasty

___ 652. cyt/o

___ 653. cutan/e

___ 654. myelin

___ 655. polymorphonuclear

___ 656. nonunion

___ 657. reflux

___ 658. 2 articulations of elbow joint

___ 659. tendin

___ 660. anorexia

___ 661. murmur

___ 662. mania

___ 663. nici

___ 664. cervic

___ 665. abduction

___ 666. closed, simple fracture

___ 667. r- integument

___ 668. diverticulum

___ 669. appendic

___ 670. prone

___ 671. phleb/o

___ 672. endoscope

___ 673. fibula

___ 674. dem

___ 675. onychomycosis

___ 676. dips

___ 677. ventral

___ 678. cyst

___ 679. clot

___ 680. myring

___ 681. hyperpyrexia

Z22. * proc of losing myelin sheath of nerve fiber

A23. any mass of tissue that projects outward

B23. r- heart

C23. narrowing of a passage

D23. (also called thrombocyte)small particle involved in clotting proc

E23. chest

F23. 2 bones joined by fibrocartilage; 2 pubic bones; greek - grow together

G23. s- process of separating

H23. s- process

I23. hypertension

J23. one who does-s

K23. sticky secretion of cells in mucous membranes (Greek) slime

L23. symptoms

M23. chemical agent that relays messages from 1 nerve cell to next

N23. substance prod a hypersensitivity (allergic) reaction

O23. absence of spontaneous respiration

P23. disease when blood is taken over by WBCs and their precursers

Q23. test to monitor brain waves, muscle tension, eye movement and oxygen levels in blood as pt sleeps

R23. r-flow

S23. inflammation of bone tissue; bone marrow infection; caused by bacteria infection like staph

T23. joints between metacarpal bones and phalanges

U23. genetic disease w/excessive viscid mucus obstructing passages

V23. normal -r

W23. fibrotic seam that forms when a wound heals; scab

X23. area of skin or mucous membrane that has been scraped off

Y23. eyelid

Z23. before meals

A24. male

B24. illium, ischium, pubis

C24. incision of intestinal wall

D24. orthopedic appliance to correct an abnormalty eg. brace **, eg. pins, plates

E24. against -p

F24. instrument to examine ear

G24. absorb excess interstitial fluid and return it to bloodstream, remove foreign chemicals, cells, and debris from tissue, 3. absorb dietary lipids from small intestine

___ 682. etiology

___ 683. bride

___ 684. cholecystitis

___ 685. malabsorption

___ 686. ischemia

___ 687. gurgit

___ 688. suct

___ 689. exocrine

___ 690. glycer

___ 691. in -s

___ 692. - c

___ 693. thenar

___ 694. factir

___ 695. dia

___ 696. dandruff

___ 697. entery

___ 698. leuk

___ 699. functions of blood

___ 700. stress fx

___ 701. reduction

___ 702. vestibule

___ 703. endoscope

___ 704. NPO

___ 705. sarcoma

___ 706. bursitis

___ 707. sphincter

___ 708. - c

___ 709. agon

___ 710. debridement

___ 711. v-tach

___ 712. aphthous

___ 713. gliding joint

___ 714. calcaneus

___ 715. palpitations

___ 716. fibrillation

___ 717. ventricle

___ 718. radi

___ 719. CF

___ 720. path

___ 721. hematoma

___ 722. dyspepsia

___ 723. ptysis

___ 724. ileostomy

H24. waxy secretion of the sebaceous glands

I24. process of -s

J24. substance in food req for normal physiol funct

K24. break or tear of any organ or body part; latin - break, fracture

L24. nose bleed

M24. abdomen

N24. artificial opening into a tubular structure; end of bowel opens into skin at a stoma; illeostomy, colostomy

O24. an organism that attaches itself to, lives on or in, and derives its nutrition from another species

P24. line -r

Q24. visual exam of interior of a joint

R24. rash characterized by reddish, silver-scaled patches; (greek) itch

S24. blood in pleural cavity

T24. stringy protein fiber; part of blood clot

U24. bone marrow is unable to prod sufficient red cells, white cells, and platelets

V24. excessive amount of sebum

W24. viscous, sticky

X24. work, activity -r

Y24. pancreatic hormone suppresses blood glucose levels and transports glucose into cells

Z24. also called rhinitis- acute inflamm of mucous membrane of nose

A25. blood vessel carrying blood toward heart

B25. malignant neoplams of primitive retinal cells

C25. malignant tumor originating in bone-producing cells

D25. triggered by fever in infants and toddlers 6 mos - 5 yrs, few dev epilepsy

E25. cancer of blood forming tissues; prod high no of leukocytes

F25. dilatation

G25. continuous positive airway pressure

H25. specialist stomach and intestines

I25. excessive levels of parathyroid hormone;

J25. r- appetite

K25. beyond -p

L25. r- air, lung

M25. paleness of skin

N25. fluid remaining after removal of blood cells and the formaton of clot

O25. cond w/abnormal, early conversion of cartilage into bone, leading to dwarfism

P25. large family of chemical substances found in many drugs,

___ 725. septum septa (pl)

___ 726. sinoatrial nodec (SA)

___ 727. crine

___ 728. pronation

___ 729. lyte

___ 730. homo

___ 731. retina

___ 732. TB

___ 733. hypoxemia

___ 734. later

___ 735. intracellular

___ 736. ancy

___ 737. ECG/EKG

___ 738. anter

___ 739. palate

___ 740. patell

___ 741. prepatellar

___ 742. fibrin

___ 743. thrombocyte, also called platelet

___ 744. malunion

___ 745. ventricular arrhythmias include

___ 746. fasc/i

___ 747. vein

___ 748. dors

___ 749. gallstone

___ 750. rupture

___ 751. bile

___ 752. ileum

___ 753. oral

___ 754. physical therapy

___ 755. umbilicus

___ 756. avian influenza

___ 757. duct

___ 758. displaced fracture

___ 759. - a

___ 760. contamination

___ 761. CA- MRSA

___ 762. COPD

___ 763. cavity

___ 764. phil

___ 765. osus

___ 766. rhonchus

hormones, and body components

Q25. r- side

R25. inflammation of stomach lining; prod symp of epigastric pain, feeling of fullness, nausea, occasional bleeding

S25. breathe -r

T25. removal of appendix by endoscope * (look up)

U25. fx does not extend completely across the bone; can be hairline, as in a stress fx in the foot when no separation of the 2 fragments

V25. medial and larger bone of forearm; latin - elbow, arm

W25. radius -r

X25. air tube from larynx to bronchi

Y25. r- cell

Z25. involuntary response to a stimulus; (latin) bend back

A26. an infection with lice

B26. r- cecum

C26. lipid, fat

D26. s- pertaining to

E26. pertaining to the chest (thorax)

F26. take care of -r

G26. condition of fungus infection in a nail

H26. cardiac output

I26. Epstein-Barr virus- common virus, member of Herpes family

J26. produce-s

K26. sacroiliac joint - joint between sacrum and ilium

L26. out of, away from -p

M26. vertebral column; or short projection from a bone

N26. sweat-r

O26. after

P26. p- below

Q26. (latin) poison

R26. calcium particle in vestibule of inner ear (ear stone)

S26. red blood cell

T26. process-s

U26. without oxygen

V26. status post

W26. to pass waste products of metabolism out of the body

X26. bird flu

Y26. situated at the side of a structure

Z26. dilation of respiratory bronchiles and alveoli

A27. ham, back of knee-r

B27. r/cf- retina of eye

C27. fx spirals around the long axis of the bone

___ 767. toxin

___ 768. mast

___ 769. pediculosis

___ 770. cutan/e

___ 771. lysis

___ 772. adenoid

___ 773. TIA

___ 774. sud

___ 775. reflex

___ 776. lateral collateral
      ligament

___ 777. brachialis

___ 778. atory

___ 779. vertebra vertebrae (pl)

___ 780. stricture

___ 781. desis

___ 782. atri

___ 783. lateral

___ 784. caries

___ 785. amount of blood in body

___ 786. NIDDM

___ 787. clavicle

___ 788. sprain

___ 789. traction

___ 790. cuticle

___ 791. stroke (CVA)

___ 792. regurgitate

___ 793. medial

___ 794. thorax

___ 795. colon

___ 796. AC

___ 797. lymphedema

___ 798. sub

___ 799. bronchiolitis

___ 800. opthalmos

___ 801. ior

___ 802. scoiosis

___ 803. agglutinate

___ 804. hemorrhoid

___ 805. gastrocnemius

___ 806. adenocarcinoma

___ 807. spin

___ 808. cruciate

___ 809. axilla

D27. buttocks-r

E27. r- suspend in a liquid

F27. when 2 bony ends of fx fail to heal together correctly

G27. inflammation of subcutaneous connective tissue

H27. extensive fibrotic liver disease *

I27. r- bile

J27. inflammation of joint(s)

K27. p - within, inside

L27. homrone secreted in stomach stim secretion of HCl and
increases gastric motility

M27. wall-r

N27. ankle -r

O27. gastroesophageal reflux disease- reflux (regurgitation) of
stomach's acid contents into esophagus

P27. r- squint

Q27. collection of 7 bones in foot that form ankle and instep;
latin - ankle

R27. above, upon -p

S27. premature ventricular contractions

T27. blood sputum

U27. p- one

V27. form of dementia; nvervecells inareas of brain assoc
w/memory and cognition are replaced by abnormal
protein clumps and tangles

W27. clot-r

X27. dissolve-s **

Y27. r-pus

Z27. death - r

A28. intravenous

B28. r- abdomen

C28. top layer of skin

D28. pert to -s

E28. surgery to repair, as far as possible, the function of a
joint; total replacement of hip joint

F28. pert to nearer the tailbone; (same as inferior, opposite of
cephalic)

G28. immature cell-s

H28. sacrum -r

I28. small-s

J28. study of structures of the body

K28. inflammation of pericardium, the covering of the heart

L28. disease-r

M28. function: transmit impulses for coordination, sensory
reception, motor actions; location- brain, spinal cord,
nerves

N28. excessive number of WBCs

___ 810. febrile seizure	O28. r- lung, air
___ 811. mucous	P28. sensation of pain-r
___ 812. stasis	Q28. without-par
___ 813. vertebra, vertebrae (pl)	R28. decreased blood volume in the body
___ 814. oste/o	S28. small fiber-r
___ 815. voluntary muscle	T28. new fibrous tissue formed during wound healing
___ 816. pineal gland	U28. inside lining of the heart
___ 817. eso	V28. p - upon, above
___ 818. ment	W28. decreased pH in blood and body tissues as result of upset metabolism (under 7.35)
___ 819. um	
___ 820. hallux valgus	X28. difficulty in nearsighted vision occurring in middle and old age
___ 821. locat	
___ 822. arthroscope	Y28. sweat, perspiration
___ 823. hyperglycemia	Z28. above, excess, excessive - p
___ 824. pub	A29. inflammation, infection
___ 825. hyperflexion	B29. general term for a scope to examine colon; specific name for organ used to examine- eg. gastroscope - endoscope to examine stomach
___ 826. paralyze	
___ 827. pleg	C29. deep furrow or cleft
___ 828. purpura	D29. movement, posture (tone), body heat, respiration, communication
___ 829. portal vein	
___ 830. uvea	E29. r - liver
___ 831. a	F29. surg removal of a lung
___ 832. exocrine	G29. radiography of vessels after injection of contrast material
___ 833. dislocation	H29. r/cf - lung
___ 834. brady	I29. a fx in which bone is broken into pieces
___ 835. nas	J29. moving Toward a center
___ 836. maximus	K29. r - small cell
___ 837. gastrin	L29. below normal levels of oxygen in tissues, gases, or blood
___ 838. papilla	M29. use of endoscope to perform examination
___ 839. atri	N29. from, out of-p
___ 840. retinopathy	O29. pert to groin **
___ 841. vasodilation	P29. substance in food required for normal physiologic function
___ 842. um	
___ 843. ia	Q29. cartilage that forms a rim around the socket of the hip joint; latin - lip-shaped
___ 844. comminuted fracture	
___ 845. physis	R29. malignant tumor orinating in connective tissue
___ 846. dysphagia	S29. r - nourish
___ 847. eu (r)	T29. gland that pro internal or hormonal subst and secretes it into bllod;
___ 848. dilation	U29. makes absorption of vit B12 happen
___ 849. spleen	V29. upset stomach
___ 850. postnatal	W29. lymph vessel carries chyle away from intestine
___ 851. CHF	X29. pert to being inside the trachea
___ 852. hiatus	Y29. sticky secretion o f cells in mucous membranes

___ 853. COPD

___ 854. autoimmune

___ 855. TIA

___ 856. cholelithotomy

___ 857. ABG

___ 858. cardiology

___ 859. hyperopia

___ 860. malignant

___ 861. neoplasm

___ 862. lacrim

___ 863. encephalitis

___ 864. angioplasty

___ 865. ectasis (r)

___ 866. ile

___ 867. crohn disease

___ 868. saliv

___ 869. liver

___ 870. acid/o

___ 871. embolus

___ 872. vascul

___ 873. derm

___ 874. peristalsis

___ 875. dia

___ 876. fiber

___ 877. WBC

___ 878. myocarditis

___ 879. secret

___ 880. pruit

___ 881. bi

___ 882. axial skeleton

___ 883. infarct

___ 884. intestin

___ 885. per

___ 886. flatus

___ 887. myringotomy

___ 888. ous

___ 889. ity

___ 890. transdermal

___ 891. proximal

___ 892. chyle

___ 893. hypoxia

___ 894. bronchus (pl - bronchi)

___ 895. radi

Z29. bend-r

A30. bone

B30. plaque- fatty deposit in the lining of an artery

C30. nourishment, food

D30. major muscle in back of lower leg (calf)

E30. pert to -s

F30. control of bleeding

G30. new-p

H30. pertaining to or nearer the head

I30. r-flow

J30. blood vessel with oxygenated blood; carries blood away
from heart

K30. region of the back and sides between the ribs and pelvis

L30. distress and dread caused by fear

M30. p - apart

N30. body-r

O30. surgical artificial opening

P30. cheekbone -r

Q30. thickening and hardening of the skin due to new collagen
formation

R30. strong membrane surrounding a bone

S30. radiographic image of selected slice of tissue

T30. result of - s

U30. substance -s

V30. shoulder bone

W30. r- on the inside

X30. loss of intellectual and metal functions -chronic,
progressive, irreversible

Y30. fx runs parallel to the long axis of the bone

Z30. icy cold -r

A31. back of the head -r

B31. stagnation in the flow of any body fluid; (greek) stying in
one place;

C31. parasite -r (greek) guest

D31. bacterial destruction of teeth; latin -dry rot

E31. expanded area at proximal and distal ends of a long bone
to prov increased surface area for attachment of
ligaments and tendons

F31. tarsal bone that articulates w/tibia to form the ankle joint;
latin - heel bone

G31. tumor, mass -s

H31. inflammation of the skin

I31. pertaining to the umbilicus (belly button, or the center of
the abdomen

J31. r- old man

___ 896. apnea

___ 897. sternum

___ 898. cellul

___ 899. insulin

___ 900. ganglion

___ 901. distal

___ 902. anemia

___ 903. laparoscope

___ 904. or

___ 905. thymus

___ 906. pan

___ 907. de

___ 908. nevus nevi (pl)

___ 909. chyme

___ 910. nosocomial

___ 911. gingivitis

___ 912. dermatology

___ 913. stomy

___ 914. conjunctiva

___ 915. tendon

___ 916. lysis

___ 917. jejenum

___ 918. articulation

___ 919. LDL

___ 920. atophy

___ 921. ataxia

___ 922. skeleton

___ 923. seborrhea

___ 924. pylor

___ 925. follicle

___ 926. cryosurgery

___ 927. quadriceps femoris

___ 928. -lus

___ 929. cephalic

___ 930. thromb

___ 931. luxate

___ 932. pulmon

___ 933. enter

___ 934. nat

___ 935. polio

___ 936. synthesis

___ 937. stridor

___ 938. virus

K31. r/cf- nerve

L31. chest -r

M31. dilation

N31. r- to blink

O31. r- stomach *

P31. situated nearest the center of the body; situated closest to the point of attachment to the body, refers to limbs

Q31. study of structure and function of cells, tissues, and organs

R31. membrane covering lungs and lining ribs in thoracic cavity

S31. poinsonous substance formed by a cell or organism;

T31. cystic fibrosis

U31. vital signs

V31. pertaining to

W31. r-abdomen

X31. use of concentrated, intense narrow beam of electromagnetic radiation for surg

Y31. sieve -r

Z31. redness-r

A32. diagnosis

B32. caused by sensitivity to gluten

C32. fecal occult blood test

D32. high BP

E32. related to the stomach **

F32. removal of injured or necrotic (dead) tissue

G32. rapid heart rate, above 100 bpm

H32. hollow at back of knee

I32. r- balance; equilibrium - equally balanced

J32. graft from another species (same as heterograft)

K32. single mass of lymph tissue in midline at back of throat

L32. nonvascular, firm connective tissue found mostly in joints; (latin) gristle

M32. end of whip

N32. wax

O32. nothing by mouth

P32. r-swallowing

Q32. spec in the structure, chemisty, and pathology of the cell

R32. bone forms part of medial wall of orbit (around eye),

S32. joint between acromion and calvicle

T32. to secrete -r

U32. p- before

V32. shortness of breath

W32. lying face up, flat on back

X32. fever blister, recurrent ulcer of lips, lining of mouth and

___ 939. glucogen

___ 940. femor

___ 941. pulmon/o

___ 942. onych/o

___ 943. urinary system

___ 944. lacrimal

___ 945. spirat

___ 946. matrix

___ 947. idiopathic

___ 948. lyt

___ 949. -ia

___ 950. temporal

___ 951. osteo

___ 952. abras

___ 953. hypovolemic

___ 954. alimentary canal

___ 955. dermatomyositis

___ 956. excoriate

___ 957. pharynx

___ 958. cyte

___ 959. sphygm/o

___ 960. glia

___ 961. opthalm

___ 962. skelet

___ 963. man

___ 964. dorsal

___ 965. dist

___ 966. osteopenia

___ 967. elle

___ 968. de

___ 969. endarterectomy

___ 970. ostomy

___ 971. ventral

___ 972. ureter

___ 973. caries

___ 974. endotracheal

___ 975. Rh

___ 976. un

___ 977. alges

___ 978. infest

___ 979. macrocyte

___ 980. orex

___ 981. deglutit

gums due to infection with herpes simplex virus type 1 (HSV-1) *

Y32. r- eye

Z32. state, condition -s

A33. fluid that has passed out of tissue or capillary as result of inflammation or injury

B33. nose

C33. r/cf - abdomen

D33. tx of obesity

E33. overstretch or tear in muscle or tendon

F33. drooping of eyelid

G33. r- suspend in liquid

H33. formed from gastronemius and soleus muscles inserted into calcaneus

I33. band of muscle that encircles an opening, when it contracts the opening squeezes closed; forms a 1 way valve

J33. surgical repair -s

K33. curved bone that forms part of the pectoral girdle

L33. joint -r

M33. disorder causing mental disruption and loss of contact w/reality

N33. severe ha,

O33. disease due to Vit D deficiency, prod soft, flexible bones; old english -to twist

P33. narrow -r

Q33. ankle -r

R33. r- lung

S33. r-intestine *

T33. potent glucocorticoidw/ antiinflammatory properties

U33. pert to lungs and their blood supply **

V33. r- eye

W33. dense, ivory-like subst located under enamel in tooth

X33. artificial opening from colon to outside of body

Y33. lubricating

Z33. r- sensation

A34. cell resulting from union of sperm and egg; (Greek) yolk

B34. r - to join; combining or blending of distinct bodies into one

C34. phalanx, finger or toe

D34. instrument for viewing retina

E34. degenerative disease of retina

F34. lymph node-r

G34. r- fully developed

H34. break down-r

___ 982. sagittal

___ 983. respir

___ 984. laparotomy

___ 985. capit/u

___ 986. dysrhythmia

___ 987. tendonitis, tendinitis

___ 988. stabismus

___ 989. steth/o

___ 990. opthamology

___ 991. CDiff

___ 992. electr/o

___ 993. rheumat

___ 994. sickle cell anemia

___ 995. metabolism

___ 996. somn (r)

___ 997. duct

___ 998. hemophilia

___ 999. systole/e

___ 1000. cutan/e

___ 1001. chir/o

___ 1002. muc/o

___ 1003. ECG, EKG,

___ 1004. epithelial tissue

___ 1005. lacteal

___ 1006. IBS

___ 1007. strab

___ 1008. mucus

___ 1009. col

___ 1010. oblique fx

___ 1011. ate

___ 1012. hypoparathyroidism

___ 1013. 4 ligaments hold knee together

___ 1014. tarsal

___ 1015. retinopathy

___ 1016. gen

___ 1017. tomy

___ 1018. isch

___ 1019. acute

___ 1020. bolus

___ 1021. CVA

___ 1022. ileus

___ 1023. coarct

___ 1024. number of bones in

I34. inflammatory connective tissue disease affecting the whole body

J34. r - away from the center

K34. to view -s

L34. radiation, xrays -r

M34. 1. maintains body's homeostasis, 2. transports nutrients, vit, and minerals,3. transports waste prod, 4. transports hormones, 5 transports gases- O2, CO2, 6. protects from foreign subs- microorganisms+toxins, 7 forms clots

N34. band of fibrous tissue connecting 2 structures; (latin) band

O34. part of vert column that forms part of the pelvis; latin - sacred

P34. an anterior thigh muscle w/4 heads (origins)

Q34. surgical incision-s

R34. reion of pharynx at back of nose and above soft pallate

S34. oxygen -r

T34. spit-r

U34. projecting forward -p

V34. mobile muscle mass in the mouth; has the taste buds *

W34. surgical removal of adipose tissue

X34. process of breathing, exchange of oxygen and carbon dioxide

Y34. disc of cartilage between bones of a joint, eg the knee joint; greek - crescent

Z34. substance, chemical compound

A35. hollow space or body compartment

B35. s - resembling

C35. within normal limits

D35. to fuse toghether

E35. visual evoked potential

F35. r- paralysis

G35. r-to swallow

H35. together -p

I35. sense of smell

J35. action -s

K35. inflamm of vein w/clot formation

L35. artificial opening from ileum to outside of body

M35. difficulty breathing

N35. wide -r

O35. acid of gastric juice

P35. presence of large numbers of specific, diagnostic mononuclear leukocytes

Q35. intramuscular

R35. r- thirst

S35. pertaining to - s

body

___ 1025. intus

___ 1026. en

___ 1027. tract

___ 1028. maxilla

___ 1029. card

___ 1030. para

___ 1031. presby

___ 1032. meniscus, menisci (pl)

___ 1033. polyp

___ 1034. resection

___ 1035. tenosynovitis

___ 1036. pyorrhea

___ 1037. metacarpophalangeal joint

___ 1038. fungus fungi (pl)

___ 1039. iron deficiency anemia

___ 1040. peri

___ 1041. dent

___ 1042. sphincter

___ 1043. ive

___ 1044. brachi/i

___ 1045. 4 knee joint bones

___ 1046. uln

___ 1047. ganglion

___ 1048. ped

___ 1049. transverse fx

___ 1050. peristalsis

___ 1051. flatul

___ 1052. silicosis

___ 1053. celiac disease

___ 1054. rhinoplasty

___ 1055. appendectomhy

___ 1056. scald

___ 1057. atic

___ 1058. seb/o

___ 1059. optometrist

___ 1060. system

___ 1061. WNL

___ 1062. CF

___ 1063. nas

___ 1064. cecum

___ 1065. NIDDM

___ 1066. polyphagia

T35. ribonucleic acid - the information carrier from DNA in the nucleus to an organelle to produce protein molecules

U35. fatigue fx caused by repetitive, local stress on a bone, as occurs in marching or running

V35. cond of having gallstones

W35. no known allergies **

X35. fibrous membrane covering a bone

Y35. when necessary

Z35. white blood cell w/o granules in cytoplasm

A36. tumor, mass -s

B36. fixed source of a muscle at its attachment to bone

C36. p- outward

D36. s- condition, action

E36. * endocrine gland in floor and wall of 3rd ventricle of Brain

F36. p- large

G36. resembling -s

H36. rod shaped

I36. r - organ; (latin) intrument, tool

J36. low density lipoprotein- bad cholesterol

K36. surgical repair of an eyelid

L36. dilated rectal vein prod painful anal swelling

M36. all-p

N36. humpbacked condition

O36. r/cf - air, lung

P36. low bp

Q36. within the cell

R36. going across or through skin

S36. class of food substances based on amino acids

T36. r- accumulation of fluid

U36. p- outward, outside

V36. chronic airway obstruction

W36. excessive production of ketones, making the blood acidic

X36. pertaining to

Y36. light rays at a higher frequency than the violet end of the spectrum

Z36. r- appendix

A37. r/cf - acid

B37. detached piece of thrombus, mass of bacteria,air, or foreign body that blocks a blood vessel

C37. r- spinal cord

D37. every

E37. p - around

F37. the population of microorganisms covering the exterior

_____ 1067. Hemoccult test

_____ 1068. hypotension

_____ 1069. chlor

_____ 1070. osteogenesis

_____ 1071. Duchenne muscular dystrophy

_____ 1072. paresis

_____ 1073. epidermis

_____ 1074. ileum

_____ 1075. glob

_____ 1076. glyc

_____ 1077. erythrocyte

_____ 1078. malacia

_____ 1079. necrosis

_____ 1080. sphen

_____ 1081. alis

_____ 1082. glutin

_____ 1083. anti

_____ 1084. stapes

_____ 1085. hypodermis

_____ 1086. path/o

_____ 1087. exo

_____ 1088. sebaceous glands

_____ 1089. gigiv

_____ 1090. pulmonary

_____ 1091. coryza

_____ 1092. shock

_____ 1093. chlor

_____ 1094. zyme

_____ 1095. sigmoid

_____ 1096. flatulence

_____ 1097. masticate

_____ 1098. dorsum

_____ 1099. ary

_____ 1100. radi/o

_____ 1101. lens

_____ 1102. rale

_____ 1103. tiz

_____ 1104. embol

_____ 1105. sacr/o

_____ 1106. 4 valves of heart

_____ 1107. transverse

_____ 1108. gastr

and interior surfaces of healthy animals; (latin) flower

G37. white

H37. synovial membrane-r

I37. correct-r

J37. func: movement; attached to bones; found in the walls of hollow tubes, organs, and the heart

K37. back of any part of body, including hand

L37. protein present in skin, hair, and nails

M37. fx runs diagonally across the long axis of the bone

N37. partial paralysis; weakness r-weakness

O37. upper part of skull that encloses and protects brain; greek -skull

P37. s - end result

Q37. s- disease

R37. mass of tissue that projects into lume of bowel *

S37. study of the lungs

T37. white-r

U37. pertaining to both sides of the body

V37. congestive heart failure

W37. surgical repair -s

X37. without -p

Y37. minute blood vessel between arterial and venous systems

Z37. alternating light and dark bands of protein filaments resp for muscle contraction; skeletal muscle - striated muscle

A38. fat

B38. surg created new opening in tympanic membrane to allow fluid to drain from middle ear (ear tubes)

C38. instrument used toexamine interior of tubular or hollow organ * (endoscope - look inside, a generic term for scope to examine)

D38. without, out of, removal, from

E38. mass of tissue that projects into lumen of bowel

F38. blowing

G38. growth plate - at ends of long bones allow for growth

H38. p- beside

I38. vein-r

J38. thymus gland -r

K38. general term used to describe yeasts and molds

L38. gland that secretes substances outwardly thru excretory ducts

M38. sore caused by lying down for long periods of time

N38. thigh bone

O38. pelvis -r

P38. inflammation of the skin and muscles

Q38. pinpoint capillary hemorrhagic spot in skin

___ 1109. gastr

___ 1110. anorexia

___ 1111. teratogen

___ 1112. pract

___ 1113. aplastic anemia

___ 1114. thym

___ 1115. hiatus

___ 1116. immunoglobulin (Ig)

___ 1117. osis

___ 1118. hypothenar eminence

___ 1119. comedo comedones (pl)

___ 1120. mi

___ 1121. pathologic fracture

___ 1122. abdomin

___ 1123. incub

___ 1124. andr/o

___ 1125. vesicle

___ 1126. ion

___ 1127. endocrine gland

___ 1128. drome

___ 1129. post

___ 1130. gener

___ 1131. ocular

___ 1132. hyperparathyroidism

___ 1133. gluteus

___ 1134. thoracic

___ 1135. mature

___ 1136. palate

___ 1137. myel

___ 1138. illium

___ 1139. prognosis

___ 1140. proctologist

___ 1141. patell

___ 1142. erg

___ 1143. xenograft

___ 1144. ligament

___ 1145. spleen functions

___ 1146. ocul

___ 1147. gall

___ 1148. py

___ 1149. hemolysis

___ 1150. hormone

___ 1151. abdomin/o

R38. cond - upper eyelid is constantly drooped over eye, due to paresis of muscle that raises upper lid

S38. 1 of 4 regions of the surface of the abdomen; 1/4 of a circle,(latin) one quarter

T38. r- eye

U38. muscular sheet separting the abdominal and thoracic cavities

V38. act of adjusting somethng to make it fit the needs

W38. head-r

X38. any disorder affecting the nervous system

Y38. WBC w/multilobed nucleus

Z38. tummy tuck; surgical removal of excess subcutaneous fat from abdominal wall

A39. stagnate, stay in one place -r

B39. instrument (endoscope) used for viewing abdominal contents *

C39. produce,create-r

D39. r-glucose, sugar

E39. metabolic syndrome caused by insulin deficiency

F39. pertaining to the stomach

G39. without

H39. with, together-p

I39. roof of the mouth , anterior 2/3 is hard palate, posterior is soft palate *

J39. inflammation of lining of heart **

K39. affect in a specific way -s

L39. pertainint to the chest

M39. study of medical imaging

N39. infection with candida albicans; occuring anywhere in mouth

O39. basin-shaped ring of bones, ligaments, and muscles at the base of the spoine

P39. forearm bone on the thumb side; latin - spoke of a wheel

Q39. new growth, benign or malignant tumor

R39. instrument-s

S39. rubbish -r

T39. situated at the side; often to bypass an obstruction

U39. structure with specific functions in the body

V39. r- middle

W39. endocrine gland in mediastinum

X39. violet, bluish-purple -r

Y39. non-insulent dependent diabetes mellitus

Z39. together -p

A40. small bone, particularly relat to 3 bones in middle ear

B40. an organ slips out of its normal position; latin-falling

___ 1152. therapy	C40. fibula -r
___ 1153. albicans	D40. free will-r
___ 1154. A+O	E40. gland that prod an internal or hormonal substance and secretes it into bloodstream
___ 1155. brachioradialis	F40. granulomatoous lesion of lungs and other organs
___ 1156. diabet	G40. infection alongside the nail
___ 1157. quadrant	H40. pert to hiatus (eg. hiatal hernia)
___ 1158. graft	I40. breathe -r
___ 1159. hypotensive	J40. s- pertaining to
___ 1160. lact	K40. skin graft from another person or cadaver
___ 1161. NPO	L40. state of hypersensitivity to an allergen - allergic
___ 1162. granulation	M40. hairlike structure-r
___ 1163. centesis (r)	N40. candida -r
___ 1164. nucleus	O40. brief but unpleasant sensations of a rapid or irregular heartbeat; caused by exercise, anxiety, stimulants (caffeine)
___ 1165. anthracosis	
___ 1166. achondroplasia	
___ 1167. podiatry	P40. r- yellow
___ 1168. epistaxis	Q40. flat, scale-like epithelial cell;(latin) scaly
___ 1169. trophy	R40. general term for all types of fatty compounds; eg. cholesterol, triglycerides, fatty acids; (Greek) fat
___ 1170. metatarsus	
___ 1171. tinea capitis	S40. excessive, excess, above, beyond -p
___ 1172. q	T40. porridge, gruel -r
___ 1173. hydrocortisone	U40. become narrow
___ 1174. leukocytosis	V40. w/o symptoms or abnormalities
___ 1175. osteomyelitis	W40. r - to breathe
___ 1176. squamous cell	X40. cartilage
___ 1177. occipital	Y40. resembling-s
___ 1178. substernal	Z40. windpipe
___ 1179. pneumon	A41. palm-r
___ 1180. triglyceride	B41. chronic obstructive pulmonary disease; use Fowlers position
___ 1181. stenosis	
___ 1182. meta	C41. substance -s
___ 1183. chondr	D41. endocrine gland in neck
___ 1184. EBV	E41. skeleton -r
___ 1185. integument, integumentary system	F41. pulley -r
	G41. extensive fibrotic liver disease
___ 1186. re	H41. to tear
___ 1187. ous	I41. central portion of a structure surrounded by cortex, contains marrow; latin - marrow
___ 1188. imus	
___ 1189. pylorus	J41. control, stop-s
___ 1190. Braden Risk Assessment scale	K41. one of bones of spinal column
	L41. crescent, meniscus -r
___ 1191. whiplash	M41. GI bleed; gastrointestinal bleed
___ 1192. dermabrasion	N41. a WBC that containes mult small granules in cytoplasm
___ 1193. de	O41. around the time of birth

___ 1194. synovial	P41. subcutaneous
___ 1195. arrhythmia	Q41. r- head pain
___ 1196. incision	R41. full of -s
___ 1197. microcyte	S41. s-pertaining to
___ 1198. ous	T41. r- normal function
___ 1199. pharynx	U41. to scratch
___ 1200. deltoid	V41. dilation of heart cavities, during which they fill w/blood
___ 1201. cervix	W41. vertical plane through the body divides it into right and left planes
___ 1202. de	X41. restoration of uncontrolled twitching of cardiac muscle fibers to normal rhythm
___ 1203. prostrate prostration (noun)	Y41. bone marrow
___ 1204. prn	Z41. s- one who studies, specialist
___ 1205. aliment	A42. inflammation of lining of esophagus *
___ 1206. osteoarthritis	B42. small, dilation of arter or cardiac chamber
___ 1207. DNRCC	C42. coronary vascular accident; stroke
___ 1208. matrix	D42. fibrous band that connects muscle to bone; latin - sinew
___ 1209. ive	E42. muscle
___ 1210. SI	F42. patella -r
___ 1211. pectoral girdle	G42. r - pelvis
___ 1212. lassissimus dorsi	H42. removal of upper layers of skin by rotary brush
___ 1213. adduction	I42. transient ischemic attack
___ 1214. ethmoid	J42. varicosity, dilated, tortuous vein-r
___ 1215. reflux	K42. electrocardiogram; record of elect signals of heart **
___ 1216. HTN	L42. a device that can be inserted into tissues
___ 1217. radiology	M42. yellow staining of tissues w/bile pigments, including bilirubin
___ 1218. pyorrhea	N42. fleshy mass at base of little finger
___ 1219. urin	O42. rotate-r
___ 1220. metabol	P42. backward flow
___ 1221. osteoblast	Q42. mass, tumor - s
___ 1222. ilium	R42. r- belly
___ 1223. prolapse	S42. disease of unknown etiology
___ 1224. mamm/o	T42. breast
___ 1225. pod	U42. all the heart muscle
___ 1226. cold sore	V42. before meals
___ 1227. gastrocnem	W42. vascular canals in bone
___ 1228. HCl	X42. puchlike opening or sac from tubular structure (eg intestine) *
___ 1229. VS	Y42. r- to lead
___ 1230. coagulant	Z42. fully developed
___ 1231. BS	A43. muscle that lies underneath biceps and is stronges flexor of forearm
___ 1232. myop	B43. s- pertaining to
___ 1233. A-fib	C43. r - nucleus
___ 1234. heterograft	
___ 1235. eupnea	
___ 1236. lyze	

___ 1237. peps	D43. Rhesus
___ 1238. empyema	E43. r- skull
___ 1239. linear fx	F43. surgical removal
___ 1240. lacer	G43. (subcutaneus) below the dermis, 3rd layer of skin, deepest layer
___ 1241. unilateral	H43. gas expelled thru anus
___ 1242. sinus	I43. to produce a chemical substance in a cell and release it from the cell
___ 1243. orthotic	J43. surgical removal of part or all of a structure
___ 1244. spir	K43. r- pylorus, gate *
___ 1245. CHD	L43. produce -r
___ 1246. cranium	M43. do not resuscitate, comfort care
___ 1247. phys	N43. 2 bones forming the side walls and roof of the cranium
___ 1248. trochlea	O43. incision into trachea to create tracheostomy
___ 1249. osteogenic sarcoma	P43. skin
___ 1250. gen	Q43. a process-s
___ 1251. ex	R43. graft removed from the patient's own skin
___ 1252. bulla	S43. s - produce, form
___ 1253. nasopharynx	T43. inflamm of tendon and its surrounding synovial sheath
___ 1254. phalanges	U43. final product of carbohydrate digestion; main sugar in blood
___ 1255. arteriosclerosis	V43. r-milk
___ 1256. diaphor	W43. pertaining to the cevix, or to the neck region
___ 1257. insul	X43. urinary tract infection
___ 1258. -ar	Y43. union of male sperm and female egg
___ 1259. tox	Z43. situated away from the center of the body;farthest from the point of attachment, refers only to limbs
___ 1260. periosteum	A44. pulseless nonbreather
___ 1261. orthopedic	B44. to flow backward, eg. blood thru a heart valve
___ 1262. eti/o	C44. inside a vein
___ 1263. lign	D44. 1 of 2 largest veins in body
___ 1264. enter	E44. immediate severe allergic response **
___ 1265. insul	F44. act of swallowing
___ 1266. isch	G44. structure -r
___ 1267. gasteroenterology	H44. electro encephalogram - record of electrical activity of brain *
___ 1268. lipid	I44. chamber where blood enters heart on both right and left sides
___ 1269. oste/o	J44. wrist bones -r
___ 1270. oste	K44. voice box
___ 1271. labrum	L44. fertilization of egg by sperm to form a zygote
___ 1272. nasolacrimal	M44. shingles; painful eruption of vesicles that follows a nerve root on one side of the body; (greek) to creep or spread
___ 1273. fertilization	
___ 1274. epiglottis	N44. r- neck
___ 1275. oma	
___ 1276. ptosis	
___ 1277. farct	
___ 1278. infarct	
___ 1279. pace	

___ 1280. allo

___ 1281. diaphragm

___ 1282. SQ, SC

___ 1283. acetaminophen

___ 1284. hip bones - 3 fused together

___ 1285. polydipsia

___ 1286. arthrocentesis

___ 1287. Lymphatic system - 3 functions

___ 1288. arthr

___ 1289. psoriasis

___ 1290. AMI

___ 1291. esthes

___ 1292. cor pulmonale

___ 1293. pre

___ 1294. pernicious anemia (PA)

___ 1295. itis

___ 1296. endo

___ 1297. an

___ 1298. kyphosis

___ 1299. gastritis

___ 1300. rrhea

___ 1301. esthes

___ 1302. opia

___ 1303. thromb

___ 1304. endocrine

___ 1305. HS

___ 1306. spina bifida

___ 1307. thrombus

___ 1308. articul

___ 1309. steroid

___ 1310. celi

___ 1311. nosocomial

___ 1312. pulmon

___ 1313. histology

___ 1314. librium

___ 1315. pharynx (pharyng-r)

___ 1316. otologist

___ 1317. hyper

___ 1318. diaphragm/a

___ 1319. crani

___ 1320. tubercul (r)

___ 1321. FX

O44. sym casued by sudden, extesion/flexion of neck

P44. center of modified cardiac muscle fibers in the wall of right atrium that acts as the pacemaker for heart rhythm

Q44. red blood cell

R44. absense of contractions of the heart

S44. joint between the temporal bone and the mandible (jaw bone joint below ear)

T44. acute rhinitis; viral inflammof mucous membrane of nose

U44. forming, pertaining to -s

V44. nourishment -r

W44. entrance, atrium -r

X44. r - box

Y44. collapse of part of lung

Z44. destruction of red blood cells so that hemoglobin is liberated

A45. s - body

B45. atrium -r

C45. chemical formed in 1 tissue or ogran and carried by blood to stim or inhiit a functin of another tissue or organ

D45. treatment -s

E45. crooked -r

F45. implantable cardioverter/defibrillator- sense abnormal rhythms; gives heart small shock to return rhythm to normal

G45. tumor, mass -s

H45. dramatic form of seizue with: loc, eyes roll up, jaw clenched, may stop breathing

I45. infant born after 42 wks gestation

J45. all-p

K45. spherical mass of cells containing a cavit or a small cul-de-sac; such as hair follicles; (latin) small sac

L45. away from -p

M45. yeastlike fungus

N45. r- lens opacity

O45. inflammation of pancreas, causes difficulty regulating insulin and sugar

P45. hematocrit- percentage of red blood cells in blood

Q45. strength of pathogen

R45. without -p

S45. per to disease of unknown etiology

T45. process of breathing; exchange of carbon dioxide and oxygen

U45. West Nile virus

V45. r- gland

W45. larynx -r

X45. spine

___ 1322. GERD	Y45. jock itch; infection of the groin
___ 1323. al	Z45. r- intestine
___ 1324. nutrient	A46. again-p
___ 1325. heart block	B46. r/cf - cell
___ 1326. poliomyelitis	C46. incomplete
___ 1327. asystole	D46. r- gut, intestine
___ 1328. oid	E46. produce
___ 1329. GIB	F46. to stick together to form clumps
___ 1330. anthrax	G46. fixation or stiffening of a joint by surgery
___ 1331. alimentary	H46. cond having gallstones (bile stones) *
___ 1332. efferent	I46. skilled in meas of vision, can't treat or pres meds
___ 1333. marrow	J46. digest tube from stomach to anus
___ 1334. spirometer	K46. cancer arising from glandualr epitheal cells; aden-gland; carcin -cancer
___ 1335. concuss	
___ 1336. trans	L46. disc of cartilage between the bones of the joint (eg. at knee cap); (latin) cresent
___ 1337. tendon	
___ 1338. serum	M46. pit in the abdomen where the umbilical cord entered the fetus
___ 1339. myc	
___ 1340. tarsus	N46. point-r
___ 1341. inguinal	O46. r-gum
___ 1342. arthr/o	P46. completely out of joint
___ 1343. stin	Q46. r-opening
___ 1344. pruritis	R46. chronic obstructive pulmonary disease; use Fowlers position
___ 1345. MRSA	
___ 1346. IM	S46. recanalization of blood vessel by surgery
___ 1347. PDA	T46. volume-r
___ 1348. constip	U46. sudden physical or mental collapse or circulatory collapse; (german) to clash
___ 1349. lip	
___ 1350. WNL	V46. small grain
___ 1351. laparoscopic appendectomy	W46. action of moving Away from midline, **
	X46. group of proteins in serum- finish off work of antibodies to destroy bacteria and other cells
___ 1352. rotator cuff tear	
___ 1353. um	Y46. abnormal heart sound heart w/stethoscope when a valve closes or opens abnormally
___ 1354. acetabulum	
___ 1355. tachypnea	Z46. r- running
___ 1356. antecubital	A47. deviation of the big toe toward the medial side of the foot (turns out)
___ 1357. melan	
___ 1358. de	B47. cut off
___ 1359. conjunctivitis	C47. laryngotracheobronchitis- infection of upper airways in children; with barking cough
___ 1360. cryo	
___ 1361. osteoporosis	D47. systematic treatment of disease, dysfunction, or disorder
___ 1362. stenosis	E47. r- maker
___ 1363. premature	F47. after the time of birth
___ 1364. muscle	G47. chest -r
	H47. r- normal function
	I47. greek - sac, bladder; abnormal fluid-filled sac such as gall

___ 1365. gastroenteritis	bladder or urinary bladder, surrounded by a membrane
___ 1366. lapar	J47. soft, flexible bones lacking in calcium - rickets
___ 1367. ary	K47. skin-r
___ 1368. ade	L47. separate - r
___ 1369. rhin	M47. consume bacteria, initiate immune response, consume old, defective erthyrocytes, serve as reservoir
___ 1370. hinge joint	N47. r-bile
___ 1371. IV	O47. restore a structure to its normal position
___ 1372. cyte	P47. central, transparent part of outer coat of eye covers iris and pupil
___ 1373. intra	Q47. purulent discharge (pus)
___ 1374. py	R47. r- seizure *
___ 1375. syncope	S47. safety reminder device; eg. soft restraint
___ 1376. fibul	T47. pulse rate
___ 1377. electrolyte	U47. fx of lower end of fibula, often w/fx of tibial malleolus; at ankle
___ 1378. commodat	V47. introduction of a substance other than blood by IV
___ 1379. URI	W47. r-mouth
___ 1380. ligament	X47. lying face down, flat on belly; (latin) bending forward
___ 1381. WNV	Y47. alert and oriented; to : purpose, time, place, person, (A+Ox1, A+Ox2,...)
___ 1382. neuropathy	Z47. r- rectum, anus *
___ 1383. fissure	A48. junction of skin and mucous membrane; (eg. the lips)
___ 1384. HDL	B48. composed of-s
___ 1385. asymptomatic	C48. destruction-s
___ 1386. proctitis	D48. clavicle -r
___ 1387. pylorus	E48. abnormal sensation - tingling, numbness, burning, prickling
___ 1388. stricture	F48. closed sac containing synovial fluid
___ 1389. blast	G48. 1 of 2 division of autonomic nerv sys operating at unconscious level
___ 1390. cec	H48. to produce, create -s
___ 1391. brachi/o	I48. blood vessel
___ 1392. atric	J48. flow-s
___ 1393. thoracotomy	K48. as needed
___ 1394. homeostasis	L48. self-p
___ 1395. sagitt	M48. artificial opening from colon to outside of body
___ 1396. pacemaker	N48. bone that forms the back of the nose and encloses numerous air cells
___ 1397. muscle tissue	O48. at the side, often to bypass an obstruction
___ 1398. paronychia	P48. narrow-r
___ 1399. emphysema	Q48. backward flow
___ 1400. etic	R48. small terminal artery leading into capillary network
___ 1401. tonic	S48. head -r
___ 1402. symptom	T48. attraction-s
___ 1403. axill	
___ 1404. fissure	
___ 1405. herni	
___ 1406. polyp	
___ 1407. SX	

___ 1408. protein

___ 1409. cruciate

___ 1410. zygote

___ 1411. endocrine

___ 1412. chondr/o

___ 1413. transfusion

___ 1414. paresthesia

___ 1415. anabolism

___ 1416. carp

___ 1417. anaphylaxis

___ 1418. labyrinth

___ 1419. my

___ 1420. septum, septa (pl)

___ 1421. haversian canals

___ 1422. prostate

___ 1423. eczema

___ 1424. varic

___ 1425. pathy

___ 1426. mucocutaneous

___ 1427. mammoplasty

___ 1428. contracture

___ 1429. impacted fx

___ 1430. abdomen

___ 1431. cardiomegaly

___ 1432. parasympathetic nervous system

___ 1433. eminence

___ 1434. stigmat

___ 1435. concussion

___ 1436. sphenoid

___ 1437. gnosis

___ 1438. re

___ 1439. allergen

___ 1440. tachy

___ 1441. physic

___ 1442. cytologist

___ 1443. trans

___ 1444. detoxification

___ 1445. physema (r)

___ 1446. patella patellae (pl)t

___ 1447. CO

___ 1448. gingiv

___ 1449. retro

___ 1450. tens

U48. sacrum -r;

V48. thin, circular bone embedded in the patellar tendon in front of the knee joint; kneecap; (latin) small plate

W48. cell that forms collagen fibers

X48. tiss surrounding teeth and covering jaw

Y48. r-chew

Z48. r- sensation

A49. ischium, hip bone -r

B49. med practice based on maintaining balance of the body

C49. r- gate, pylorus

D49. bend down-r

E49. to swing

F49. draw -r

G49. cell

H49. pancreatic hormone that suppresses blood glucose levels and transports glucose into cells

I49. a bone is broken into at least 2 fragments

J49. red blood cell condition where number of RBCs or amt of hemoglobin in q RBC is reduced

K49. r- flatus, excessive gas

L49. high pitched noise made when respir obstruction in larynx or trachea

M49. fluid filled cyst on back of wrist, result from irritation or inflamm of synovial tendon sheaths

N49. causes warts and is associated with cancer

O49. before expected time, eg infant born before 37 wks gestation

P49. hormone present in many tissues, but first isolated from prostate gland

Q49. process of recording

R49. material of sheat around axon of a nerve

S49. subcutaneous

T49. operate-r

U49. relating to stomach and duodenum

V49. stationary-r

W49. body in the nucleus that contains DNA and genes

X49. crooked condition of spine

Y49. r -diabetes

Z49. rapid breathing, over 24/minute

A50. basic building blocks of protein

B50. r- destroy

C50. skin

D50. skeleton

E50. 22 - 8 cranial, 14 facial

F50. 3rd portion of the small intestine (Latin) to twist or roll

___ 1451. ectasis (r)

___ 1452. bunion

___ 1453. oma

___ 1454. tendinitis (also spelled tendonitis)

___ 1455. contract

___ 1456. glucose

___ 1457. ana

___ 1458. atri

___ 1459. vetebral column - how many bones

___ 1460. plasma

___ 1461. Ig

___ 1462. osteomalacia

___ 1463. angiogram

___ 1464. scapula , scapulae (pl)

___ 1465. olfaction, olfact (r)

___ 1466. ventr

___ 1467. incubation

___ 1468. pneumoconiosis

___ 1469. bradycardia

___ 1470. wheal

___ 1471. cardi/o

___ 1472. macrocytic

___ 1473. quadriplegia

___ 1474. granulocyte

___ 1475. stat

___ 1476. fibroblast

___ 1477. accomodation

___ 1478. burs

___ 1479. afferent

___ 1480. cirrhosis

___ 1481. popliteal fossa

___ 1482. palpat

___ 1483. peri

___ 1484. trochle

___ 1485. pubis

___ 1486. surg

___ 1487. candidiasis

___ 1488. cartilage

___ 1489. organelle

___ 1490. synthetic

___ 1491. ism

___ 1492. mature

up

G50. funct - bind, support, protect, fill spaces, store fat; found throughout body (eg. blood, bone cartilage, and fat

H50. before, in front of -p

I50. lymphoma- chronic enlargement of lymph nodes spreading to other nodes in orderly way

J50. skin-r

K50. p - across, through

L50. the vertebral column, or a short bony projection

M50. corticosteroid prod in small amounts by adrenal cortex

N50. surg spe in disease of anus and rectum

O50. artificial opening

P50. a partial fx; one side breaks, the other bends (tib/fib and radius/ulna)

Q50. tissue consisting of cells that can contract

R50. science of blood flow thru circulatio

S50. sore -r

T50. small vein leading from capillary network

U50. the process of building a compound from different elements

V50. small WBC w/large nucleus

W50. pertaining to the skin

X50. atrial fibrilallation-

Y50. supporting tissue of the body

Z50. cell receives light and converts it into electrical impulses

A51. symptoms

B51. abdominal region above the stomach

C51. dx, tx, and prevention of mechanical disorders of the musculoskeletal sys

D51. nitrogen-containing substance -s

E51. atrial septal defect

F51. artificail opening into a tubular structure

G51. outer portion of an organ, such as bone

H51. pert to mouth

I51. vital signs

J51. 1.PVC's -premature ventricular contractions, 2. v-fib- ventricular fibrillation,

K51. transport: oxygen, CO2, and nitric oxide

L51. able to see distant objects but unable to see close ** (farsighted)

M51. small, flat spot or patch on the skin; (latin) spot

N51. r- tear

O51. restoration of a normal heart rhythm by electric shock

P51. apart, away from -p

Q51. black pigment found in skin, hair, and retina

___ 1493. glauc

___ 1494. thoracentesis

___ 1495. tax

___ 1496. spiral fx

___ 1497. sis

___ 1498. bradypnea

___ 1499. ion

___ 1500. al

___ 1501. hemostasis

___ 1502. ure

___ 1503. ventr

___ 1504. phlor

___ 1505. cataract

___ 1506. humerus

___ 1507. infect

___ 1508. AP

___ 1509. phalang/e

___ 1510. crete

___ 1511. oste

___ 1512. muscul

___ 1513. lymphadenectomy

___ 1514. pro

___ 1515. infusion

___ 1516. cranium

___ 1517. constric

___ 1518. hypothyroidism

___ 1519. ery

___ 1520. avascular

___ 1521. arthr

___ 1522. nervous tissue

___ 1523. intussusception

___ 1524. deglutition

___ 1525. capill

___ 1526. neurology

___ 1527. Alzheihmer disease

___ 1528. seratonin

___ 1529. poster

___ 1530. mandibul

___ 1531. esophagitis

___ 1532. parietal

___ 1533. necrotizing fasciitis

___ 1534. ism

___ 1535. tom/o (r)

R51. endoscope used to exam interior of joint

S51. excision (cutting out) of all or part of meniscus (disc of cartilage between the bones of a joint, as in knee joint

T51. tendon-r

U51. inflammation of lung parenchyma tissue

V51. tube that connects kidney to urinary bladder, (Greek) urinary canal, passage of urine

W51. s- pertaining to

X51. lethal-r

Y51. r - navel (belly button)

Z51. touch -r (as in contagious)

A52. r- mind

B52. dilated, tortuous veins (varicose)

C52. state of -s

D52. nodule, swelling, TB

E52. globe-r

F52. r- apart from

G52. bone that forms the hard palate and parts of the nose and orbits

H52. built up or put together from simpler compounds

I52. r- digestion

J52. following a meal

K52. windpipe; 1 of 2 subdiv. of trachea

L52. proc of lying face upward, or of turning a hand or foot so that the palm or sole is facing up

M52. head-r

N52. lobulated exocrine gland, head is tucked into curve of duodenum, prod insulin

O52. detached piece of thrombus, a mass of bacteria, quantity of air, or foreign body that blocks a blood vessel

P52. regon of pharynx below the epiglottis that includes the larynx

Q52. r-green

R52. r- nitrogen containing

S52. black pigment -r

T52. between ventricles of the heart

U52. excessive gas in stomach/intestines

V52. lipid containing 3 fatty acids

W52. pressure-r

X52. presence of persecutory delusions

Y52. p- below

Z52. r- chew

A53. use of liquid nitrogen or argon gas in a probe to freeze and kill abnormal tissue

B53. p- around

___ 1536. hallux	C53. freq injury to shoulder girdle, caused by wear and tear from overuse
___ 1537. external fixation	D53. joint -r
___ 1538. ic	E53. pituitary gland, pineal gland, thyroid gland, 4 parathyroid glands, thymus, 2 adrenal glands, pancreas
___ 1539. prosthesis	F53. heart
___ 1540. muscle	G53. urine -r
___ 1541. ation	H53. sweet, glycerol-r
___ 1542. infestation	I53. fx occurring at a site already weakened by disease process, such as cancer
___ 1543. uterus	J53. athlete's foot
___ 1544. inter atrial	K53. flesh -r
___ 1545. DI - diabetes insipius	L53. plug-r
___ 1546. ket/o	M53. removing poison from a tissue or substance
___ 1547. cecum	N53. (Greek) a swelling or knot
___ 1548. arthro/o	O53. without oxygen; absence of spontaneous respiration
___ 1549. neurotransmitter	P53. r-fall in drops
___ 1550. laceration	Q53. clot attached to a diseased blood vessel or heart lining **
___ 1551. RNA	R53. ability to see objects as they come into the outer edges of visual field
___ 1552. monocyte	S53. suck
___ 1553. percutaneous	T53. nail
___ 1554. gnosis	U53. p- from ribose, a sugar
___ 1555. ectomy	V53. r- vein
___ 1556. seizure types	W53. skull
___ 1557. acne	X53. without-p
___ 1558. reflux	Y53. small sac containing liquid (eg. a blister)latin-blister
___ 1559. cilium (cilia-pl)	Z53. formative portion of a hair, nail, or tooth
___ 1560. digest	A54. larynx- throat
___ 1561. vita	B54. invade -r
___ 1562. viscos (r)	C54. cerebral hemispheres
___ 1563. symphysis	D54. fibrotic lung disease caused by inhalation of different dusts
___ 1564. adip	E54. 2 separate bones have formed a joint
___ 1565. arthritis	F54. infection of many hair follicles in asmall area, often on the back of the neck; ingrown hair
___ 1566. pept	G54. consume
___ 1567. hiatal	H54. blood vessell -r
___ 1568. periton	I54. r - back part
___ 1569. oid	J54. ventricular septal defect
___ 1570. exo	K54. p- rapid
___ 1571. hormone	L54. r-unknown
___ 1572. endocrine system	M54. w/o appetite, an aversin to food
___ 1573. later	N54. nonvascular, firm connective tissue found mostly in joints; latin - gristle
___ 1574. gasteroenterology	
___ 1575. lacteal	
___ 1576. pernicious anemia (PA)	
___ 1577. attenu	
___ 1578. rhabd/o	

____ 1622. con

____ 1623. perforation

____ 1624. po

____ 1625. caudal

____ 1626. endo

____ 1627. cystic fibrosis

____ 1628. varix, adj- varicose

____ 1629. capitulum

____ 1630. post mature

____ 1631. glucagon

____ 1632. respiration

____ 1633. tachycardia

____ 1634. external manipulation

____ 1635. atheroma

____ 1636. cholelithiasis

____ 1637. diverticulum, pl- diverticula

____ 1638. cervical

____ 1639. nasopharynx

____ 1640. myos

____ 1641. secrete

____ 1642. tomography

____ 1643. syn

____ 1644. 4 components of skeletal sys

____ 1645. sten/o

____ 1646. defibrilation

____ 1647. paresis

____ 1648. intra

____ 1649. scar

____ 1650. therap

____ 1651. alveol

____ 1652. protaglandin

____ 1653. membrane

____ 1654. tinea corporis

____ 1655. lacrim

____ 1656. lysis

____ 1657. lymphaden

____ 1658. eal

____ 1659. TMJ - temporomandibular joint

____ 1660. pedicul

____ 1661. disciplin

Z55. bone

A56. skin-r

B56. infection of the skin prod thick, yellow crusts

C56. fluid containing swelling attached to synovial sheath of a tendon

D56. * any disorder of nervous sys

E56. hemolytic disease of newborn (HDN)

F56. s- process, condition

G56. surg excis of lymph nodes

H56. pertaining to the belly or situated nearer the face of the belly

I56. 5 bones between the carpus and fingers

J56. tibia -r

K56. part of a cell having specialized function

L56. action of moving toward the midline **

M56. bursa -r

N56. process-p

O56. act of being invaded on the skin by a troublesome other species, such as a parasite

P56. different -p

Q56. surg remov of thymus gland

R56. hinge joint - humerus and ulna- allows flexion and extension of elbow; gliding joint between humerus and radius of forearm - allows pronation and supination

S56. coronary vascular accident; stroke

T56. inner ear

U56. separation of normally joined parts; greek - separation

V56. r-yellow

W56. tumor that invades surrounding tissues and metastasizes to distant organs

X56. of the arm -r

Y56. urinary tract infection

Z56. * disorder of multiple motor and vocal tics

A57. paralysis of all 4 limbs

B57. study of the cell

C57. inner (medial) one of 3 ossicles of middle ear, shaped like a stirrup

D57. agent that produces fetal deformities (eg. thalidomide)

E57. to chew

F57. pert to disease of unknown origin

G57. lack of blood supply to a tissue

H57. abnormal softness -s

I57. gluteus minimus is smallest of gluteal muscles and lies under the gluteus medius

J57. p- above

___ 1662. pathy

___ 1663. chyme

___ 1664. lymphangi

___ 1665. ICD

___ 1666. tympanostomy

___ 1667. diastasis

___ 1668. tricuspid

___ 1669. pelv

___ 1670. mastic

___ 1671. incis

___ 1672. endoscopy

___ 1673. thrombophlebitis

___ 1674. odont

___ 1675. ceps

___ 1676. chole

___ 1677. spine

___ 1678. glycogen

___ 1679. keloid

___ 1680. ion

___ 1681. Hct

___ 1682. IBS

___ 1683. com

___ 1684. ischemia

___ 1685. analgesic

___ 1686. - p

___ 1687. therapy

___ 1688. necr/o

___ 1689. function of RBC's

___ 1690. subluxation

___ 1691. papule

___ 1692. re

___ 1693. tone

___ 1694. - p

___ 1695. anoxia

___ 1696. halit

___ 1697. mononucleosis

___ 1698. hepat

___ 1699. RBC

___ 1700. PDT

___ 1701. pulmonology

___ 1702. id

___ 1703. flora

___ 1704. collagen

K57. segement of small intestine between duodenum and ileum

L57. acid of gastric juice

M57. p-back

N57. r- provide a mouth

O57. condition -s

P57. surgical removal of gallstones *

Q57. severe acute respiratory syndrome

R57. automatic external defibrillator- send electric shock to heart in order to stop the heart temporarily so tha a normal contraction rhythm can resume

S57. r-tooth

T57. lung-r

U57. osteoartritis

V57. blood group system; type A blood - has only antigen A, type B- has only antigen B, type O-has neither antigen, type AB - has antigen A and B

W57. poison -r

X57. congenital heart disease

Y57. tears -r

Z57. fleshy mass at base of thumb

A58. other-p

B58. dx and tx of diseases of eye

C58. to breathe -r

D58. thin layer of tissue covering a structure or cavity; (latin) parchment

E58. intestinal obstruction *

F58. fainting; temporary loc and postural tone due to diminshed cerebral blood flow

G58. converted by HCl in stomach to pepsin

H58. instruction -r

I58. funct: protect, secrete, absorb, excrete; location- covers body surface, covers and lines internal organs, composes glands

J58. r- coordination

K58. gran mal, petit mal, febrile

L58. wedge -r

M58. instrument used to meas respiratory volumes

N58. clot-r

O58. outer layer of the heart wall **

P58. increased intraocular pressure

Q58. fear of light because it hurts eyes

R58. hormone produced by islet cells of pancreas

S58. breakdown of food into elements suitable for cell metabolism

T58. alignment of fx by immobil bone by plaster casts, splints,

____ 1705. ment

____ 1706. nucleolus

____ 1707. jaundice

____ 1708. bicuspid

____ 1709. hypoxia

____ 1710. tinea

____ 1711. sebum

____ 1712. sclera

____ 1713. Pott fx

____ 1714. hypo

____ 1715. larnyx

____ 1716. iris

____ 1717. eustachian tube

____ 1718. compression fx

____ 1719. opthalmoscope

____ 1720. pulmonologist

____ 1721. melan

____ 1722. choledocholithisis

____ 1723. typan

____ 1724. dx

____ 1725. celi

____ 1726. ceps

____ 1727. cyst

____ 1728. thenar eminence

____ 1729. chiropractic

____ 1730. cardi/o

____ 1731. oxy

____ 1732. EEG

____ 1733. flux

____ 1734. ulna

____ 1735. flammat

____ 1736. cochlea

____ 1737. supination

____ 1738. IDDM

____ 1739. eschar

____ 1740. mutation

____ 1741. logy

____ 1742. or (os)

____ 1743. virulence

____ 1744. cranial

____ 1745. HCl - hydrochloric acid

____ 1746. spir (r)

____ 1747. leukopenia

traction or external fixators (pins, plates, halo)

U58. p- inward

V58. (pert to stomach and duodenum) in stomach and duodenum when mucosal lining breaks down

W58. with, together - p

X58. hard mass of cholseterol, calcium, and billirubin that can be formed in gb and bile duct

Y58. destruction

Z58. pert to chest **

A59. partition -r

B59. slippery lubricant stored in the joint cavity; makes joint movement almost friction free

C59. * inflammation of brain cells and tissues; brain swelling causes tissue damage

D59. scales in hair from shedding of the epidermis

E59. vertical plane dividing body into anterior and posterior portions

F59. wheezing sound heard on auscultation of lungs; made by air passing thru constricted lumen

G59. examination of contents of abdomen using an endoscope *

H59. normal posterior curve of spine that can be exaggerated in disease

I59. immunoglobulin

J59. r- nearest to the center

K59. fibrotic lung disease from inhaling silica particles

L59. r-island

M59. alert and oriented; to : purpose, time, place, person, (A+Ox1, A+Ox2,...)

N59. inflammation of a tendon

O59. blood that can't be seen in stool but is pos on feal occult blood test

P59. involving health care providers from omore than one profess

Q59. nonsteroidal anti-inflammatory drug

R59. Clostridium Difficile - very contageous diahhrea; contact isolation - gown,gloves

S59. area of dead tissue

T59. radiograph obtained after injection of radiopaque contrast material into blood vess

U59. large, fan-shaped muscle conn scapula and clavicle to humerus

V59. shaped like a cross;

W59. humrus and ulna - at elbow

X59. to form -r; as suffix - something formed

Y59. black pigment -r

Z59. a clot attached to a diseased blood vessel or heart lining

____ 1748. tonsil

____ 1749. arteriole

____ 1750. ase

____ 1751. Hgb or Hb

____ 1752. p

____ 1753. alges

____ 1754. in

____ 1755. cav

____ 1756. multi

____ 1757. dementia

____ 1758. gluc

____ 1759. follicle

____ 1760. gastritis

____ 1761. acromi

____ 1762. insert

____ 1763. myoglobin

____ 1764. papilla

____ 1765. pericarditis

____ 1766. dopamine

____ 1767. proxim

____ 1768. carpus

____ 1769. ganglion cyst

____ 1770. histamine

____ 1771. brachi

____ 1772. prothrombin

____ 1773. lymphocyte

____ 1774. lip

____ 1775. agranulocyte

____ 1776. candida

____ 1777. nici

____ 1778. fetiliz

____ 1779. aden (r)

____ 1780. ment

____ 1781. exophthalmos

____ 1782. gastric

____ 1783. lateral

____ 1784. xeno

____ 1785. ator

____ 1786. jejun

____ 1787. cec

____ 1788. laparoscopy

____ 1789. duoden

____ 1790. v-fib

A60. able to see close objects but unable to see distant; nearsighted

B60. weight -r

C60. organelles that generate, store, and release energy for cell activities

D60. calf of leg-r

E60. joint -r

F60. weaken-r

G60. patholic compression of an organ, such as the heart

H60. only gland that is both an endocrine and exocrine gland; secretes digestive juices and the hormones insulin and glucagon

I60. pull together -r

J60. surgically made union between 2 tubular structures *

K60. s- pertaining to

L60. Methicillin Resistant Stapholococus Aureus- extremely virulent staph infection, can be fatal; use contact isolation - gloves and gown

M60. s- pertaining to

N60. passage from lacrimal sac to nose

O60. s - soluble

P60. leaf shaped plate of cartilage that shuts off the larynx during swallowing

Q60. lung disease caused by inhalation of coal dust

R60. disease w/diarrhea, bowel spasms, fever, and dehydration

S60. after, subsequent to - p

T60. enzyme prod by stomach that breaks down protein

U60. dx and tx of disorders and injuries of foot

V60. deep vein thrombosis

W60. fx occurs in a vetebra from trauma or pathology, leading to the vertebra being crushed

X60. breakdown of complex substances into simpler ones as a part of metabolism

Y60. inflammatory disease of sebaceous glands and hair follicles; (greek) point

Z60. r- condition of intestine

A61. proc of lying face down on belly position, or turning a hand or foot with volar (palm or sole) surface down

B61. bad cavity; bacterial destruction of teeth

C61. reshaping by surger -s

D61. r- saliva

E61. r- secrete

F61. strength of pathogen

G61. tissue swelling due to lyphatic obstruction; differs from regular edema

H61. papilla, pimple -r

___ 1791. ganglion	I61. disease
___ 1792. rectum	J61. death
___ 1793. hemoptysis	K61. failure of one or more vertebral arches to close during fetal development
___ 1794. VS	L61. white of eye
___ 1795. colles fx	M61. a gland that produces an internal or hormonal substance
___ 1796. corticosteroid	N61. large WBC w/ single nucleus
___ 1797. papillomavirus	O61. acromioclavicular- lateral end of the scapula, extending over the shoulder joint; at end of clavicle
___ 1798. laser surgery	P61. 26
___ 1799. derma	Q61. is under control of the will
___ 1800. phagia	R61. thin wall dividing 2 cavities **
___ 1801. enzyme	S61. condition -s
___ 1802. ose	T61. r-cecum
___ 1803. metacarpals	U61. r-nourishment
___ 1804. minimus	V61. inflamm of lining of stomach
___ 1805. esophageal varices	W61. Clostridium Difficile - very contageous diahhrea; contact isolation - gown,gloves
___ 1806. cephal	X61. flood-r
___ 1807. villus, villi (pl)	Y61. invasion of the body by disease-prod microorganisms
___ 1808. MI	Z61. cervical -7, thoracic - 12, lumbar -5, sacral -1, coccyx -1
___ 1809. fibrill	A62. s- enzyme
___ 1810. papill/o	B62. the constantly changing physical and chemical rocesses occurring in the cell that are the sum of anabolism and catabolism
___ 1811. dilat	C62. subdivision of an organ or other part
___ 1812. co	D62. dislocate -r
___ 1813. cortisone	E62. transparent refractive struc behind iris
___ 1814. cytology	F62. infection w/Candida albicans; yeast infection/fungus in mouth *
___ 1815. gen	G62. acromion -r
___ 1816. respir	H62. pert to eye
___ 1817. rheumatism	I62. med spec of stomach and intestines *
___ 1818. electr/o	J62. neck region
___ 1819. cardioversion	K62. illium -r
___ 1820. latiss	L62. gland that secretes sust outwardly thru excretory ducts
___ 1821. scoli	M62. deficient levels of parathyroid hormone;
___ 1822. thrush	N62. joint -r
___ 1823. nucle	O62. p-complete
___ 1824. nutrit	P62. draw together or shorten
___ 1825. an	Q62. opening through a structure
___ 1826. idi/o	R62. inadequated GI absorption of nutrients * (causes- ciliac and crons disease)
___ 1827. iatr	S62. crackle hear thru stethoscope due to fluid in lungs, French - rattle
___ 1828. abdominoplasty	
___ 1829. DIFF	
___ 1830. lipase	
___ 1831. parotid	
___ 1832. laryng	
___ 1833. pelv	

___ 1834. supine	T62. small particle involved in clotting proc
___ 1835. kyph	U62. pertaining to respiration (breathing)
___ 1836. amblyopia	V62. ringworm infections of the body's skin and hands
___ 1837. leukemia	W62. finger or toe bones; 14 phalanges of hand- each finger has 3 joints except thumb which has only 2
___ 1838. palpitation	
___ 1839. blepharoptosis	X62. palate-r
___ 1840. pleura	Y62. side
___ 1841. dermat/o	Z62. passage of black, tarry stools
___ 1842. cor	A63. specialist for intestines
___ 1843. amino acid	B63. cut out
___ 1844. rheumatoid arthritis	C63. * sharpness and clearness of vision
___ 1845. sub	D63. pertaining to the cranium (skull)
___ 1846. diabetes mellitus	E63. the bony framework of the body
___ 1847. cervic	F63. widest (broadest) muscle in back, the "V" **
___ 1848. attenuate	G63. * tube connects middle ear to nasopharynx
___ 1849. cyst	H63. scrape off
___ 1850. thyroid	I63. r/cf - electricity
___ 1851. chromosome	J63. history and physical
___ 1852. granul	K63. canker sores
___ 1853. mandibul	L63. nose -r
___ 1854. caud	M63. cortex -r
___ 1855. blephar	N63. endocrine gland in floor an dwall of 3rd ventricle of brain; secretes feel-good hormone serotonin by day and converts it to melatonin at night
___ 1856. epiphyseal plate	
___ 1857. tag	
___ 1858. synapse	O63. fluid secreted by liver into duodenum
___ 1859. intrinsic factor	P63. normal (optimal) heart rhythm arising from SA node (sinoatrial)
___ 1860. inflammation	
___ 1861. pneumonia	Q63. having a particular quality -s
___ 1862. nasopharynx	R63. exam of contents of abdomen using endoscope
___ 1863. aden	S63. fiber-r
___ 1864. lupus	T63. r- chest
___ 1865. organ	U63. surgicqally made union between 2 tubular structures
___ 1866. DNA	V63. hormone formed by pineal gland helps regulate sleep and wake cycles
___ 1867. hypogastric	
___ 1868. mucosa	W63. r - head
___ 1869. hemothorax	X63. infection with yeastlike fungus
___ 1870. hemodynamics	Y63. combin of signs and symptoms assoc w/ a parti disease proc
___ 1871. alveolus	
___ 1872. an	Z63. make incapable of movement
___ 1873. intramuscular	A64. immature cell
___ 1874. crani	B64. r- to take up
___ 1875. demyelination	C64. narrowing of a tube
___ 1876. sacrum	D64. blind pouch that is 1st part of large intestine
	E64. substance capable of triggering an immune response
	F64. little, small -s

___ 1877. blepharitis	G64. hour of sleep; bedtime
___ 1878. macro	H64. cavity or hollow space in bone or other tissue
___ 1879. decubitus ulcer	I64. slow heart rate, less than 60 bpm
___ 1880. hyper	J64. includes: vertebral column, skull, rib cage; protects brain, spinal cord, heart, lungs
___ 1881. ab	K64. connective tissue that holds a structure together
___ 1882. oma	L64. a malignant and invasive epithelial tumor
___ 1883. vena cava	M64. r- treatment
___ 1884. insertion	N64. digestive tract
___ 1885. auto	O64. breathe
___ 1886. CVA	P64. p- without
___ 1887. rhinitis	Q64. condition -s
___ 1888. endemic	R64. insoluble protein in wheat, barley, oats
___ 1889. rhin	S64. r- hormone
___ 1890. bari	T64. plug-r
___ 1891. tendon	U64. moving away from a center
___ 1892. stalsis	V64. collar bone
___ 1893. virulence	W64. across, through -p
___ 1894. gluten	X64. hairlike motile projection from surf of cell; latin -eyelash
___ 1895. respiratory	Y64. r - join together
___ 1896. petechia	Z64. r-mandible
___ 1897. pector	A65. pain-s
___ 1898. endo	B65. throat-r
___ 1899. arthrography	C65. wasting away or diminished volume of tissue, an organ, or a body part **
___ 1900. myocardium	D65. re knee - 2 internal ligaments of knee joint cross over each other to form an "x"; latin -cross
___ 1901. rickets	E65. partial paralysis
___ 1902. necrosis	F65. tuberculosis
___ 1903. femur	G65. s- stimulation
___ 1904. excision	H65. enzyme that breaks down fat
___ 1905. a	I65. tendon-r
___ 1906. pneumonectomy	J65. incision thru chest wall
___ 1907. ical	K65. persistent, long-term disease
___ 1908. ation	L65. junction between 2 nerve cells, or a nerve fiber and its target cell, where electrical impulses are transmitted between cells
___ 1909. coll/a	M65. part of trunk between thorax and pelvis
___ 1910. graphy	N65. cond when heart rhythm is abnormal
___ 1911. hepat	O65. r- stomach
___ 1912. retin/o	P65. deoxyribonucleic acid- source of hereditary characteristics found in chromosomes
___ 1913. ation	Q65. cause
___ 1914. ease	R65. inflamm of gallbladder
___ 1915. perforation	S65. hormone secreted in stomach tath stim secretion of HCl
___ 1916. autonomic nervous system	
___ 1917. sinus rhythm	
___ 1918. enter	
___ 1919. laparascopy	

___ 1920. jejunum

___ 1921. candid

___ 1922. nerv

___ 1923. scler/o

___ 1924. lymph

___ 1925. mastic

___ 1926. scopy

___ 1927. polysomnography

___ 1928. stasis

___ 1929. an

___ 1930. venule

___ 1931. diabetes mellitus

___ 1932. stent

___ 1933. dermatitis

___ 1934. striations

___ 1935. rrhea

___ 1936. PVC's -premature ventricular contractions-

___ 1937. pan

___ 1938. thymectomy

___ 1939. thorac

___ 1940. tars

___ 1941. esophogus

___ 1942. peptic ulcer

and increases gastric motility

T65. irritable bowel syndrome

U65. high blood glucose level, over 110

V65. white blood cell

W65. incision in typanic membrane

X65. artificial opening from ileum to outside of body

Y65. small protuberance on the skin containing pus

Z65. flat-r

A66. after

B66. medial collateral ligament, lateral collateral ligament, ACL- anterior cruciate ligament, PCL - posterior cruciate ligament

C66. sudden onset

D66. entrance-r

E66. lower jaw bone

F66. ulna -r

G66. hand

H66. difficulty swallowing *

I66. r-tongue

J66. liver

K66. to chew *

L66. protein that induces changes in other substances

M66. area of cell death from infarction

N66. inner lining of eyelids

O66. fractured bone parts are out of line

P66. artifical part to remedy a defect in body **

Q66. fat-r

R66. form of skin cancer seen in AIDS patients

S66. skin

T66. p- apart

U66. transfer of blood or blood component from a donor to recipient

V66. 206

W66. r- side

X66. virus w/RNA core

Y66. breathe

Z66. pulse-r

A67. destruction of red blood cells so hemoblobin is released

B67. s- condition

C67. r- bore through

D67. middle-p

E67. transplant

F67. r- spinal cord

G67. narrowing and thickening of terminal small bowel

H67. bad, difficult -p

I67. removes waste from blood, maintains water and electrolyte balance, stores and transports urine; ureters, urethra, urinary bladder, kidneys

J67. cystic fibrosis -

K67. black pigment found in skin, hair, and the retina

L67. cancer -r

M67. bony lump on terminal phalanx of fingers in osteoartritis

N67. process to dev an infection

O67. r - change

P67. backward-p

Q67. ultraviolet

R67. r- pressure

S67. fracture

T67. big toe -r

U67. step-r

V67. 6 liters

W67. deficient prod of thyroid hormone; decreases body's metabolism

X67. nose

Y67. r/cf - color

Z67. tumor, mass-s

A68. touch, stroke-r

B68. life - r

C68. a thin wall separting 2 cavities or tissue masses

D68. arm-r

E68. vascular lymph organ in LUQ of abdomen

F68. r- stomach

G68. buildup of complex substances in the cell from simpler ones as a part of metabolism

H68. device that regulates cardiac electrical

I68. trans ischemic attack - mini stroke

J68. rupture; protrusion of structure thru tiss that normally contains it

K68. circumscribed dilation of an artery or cardiac chamber

L68. r - build up

M68. bend backward -r

N68. air sac -r

O68. r - crown

P68. nosebleed

Q68. to organize, arrange -r

R68. slow

S68. r- constrict

T68. low blood glucose level; under 70

U68. anemia due to low iron in blood

V68. deep furrow or cleft

W68. knowledge -r

X68. r-symptom

Y68. arterial blood gas

Z68. time; temple-r

A69. r- destruction

B69. r-ileum

C69. r- mind

D69. hepatitus A, B, C virus

E69. organ in which an egg develops into fetus; (latin) womb

F69. child -r

G69. blood sugar, breath sounds, bowel sounds

H69. visual examination of interior of a joint

I69. rubbish -r

J69. lethal

K69. specific protein evoked by an antigen; all antibodies are immunoglobulins

L69. enzyme that breaks down food *

M69. before

N69. flame

O69. hemoglobin-red pigmented protein; main component of red blood cells

P69. on right -tricuspid and pulmonary, on left - mitral (bicuspid) and aortic

Q69. r-pus

R69. dilated, tortuous veins in esohagus- bleed - can cause death

S69. narrowing and thickening of terminal samll bowell

T69. exit area of stomach

U69. presence of infectious agent on any surface

V69. within - p

W69. r- sight

X69. into -p

Y69. narrowing of a canal or passage; eg. of a heart valve

Z69. located in the dermis that open into hair follicles and secrete a waxy fluid called sebum

A70. foot -r

B70. non-insuline dependent diabetes mellitus, type 2 diabetes

C70. a bone-maintaing cell

D70. inability to focus light rays that enter the eye in different planes

E70. protein-r

F70. insuline dependent diabetes mellitus; type 1 diabetes,

G70. inflammation of eyelid

H70. pathologice death of cells or tissue; greek -death

I70. lead -r

J70. chronic bran disorder due to paroxysmal excessive
neuronal discharges (seizures) *

K70. protected from

L70. bone -r

M70. r-pancreas

N70. surg removal of appendix

O70. to block,

P70. skin

Q70. most common bacterium to invade the skin

R70. change in chemistry of a gene

S70. r- adjust

T70. * sudden, involuntary, repeated contraction of muscles

U70. removal of injured or necrotic tissue

V70. deficient -s

W70. lie on, hatch-r

X70. EENT -ear, nose, throat med specialist

Y70. chest x-ray

Z70. systemic disease affecting many joints

A71. persistent erythematous (redness) of the central face

B71. containing fat

C71. r- eyelid *

D71. skin

E71. p- within

F71. detailed plan; as for a regimen of therapy; (latin) contents
page of a book

G71. r- glycogen, sugar

H71. skin-r

I71. incomplete bony ring tht attaches the upper limb to the
axial skeleton; Old eng - girdle

J71. r- shake or jar

K71. kidney

L71. acute inflammation of nasal mucosa

M71. fungus

N71. forcible, rapid beat of the heart felt by patient

O71. put together -r

P71. p- within

Q71. widen, open up -r

R71. analgesic and antipyetic (pain and fever)

S71. iron-based part of hemoglobin, carries oxygen

T71. piece of detached blood clot (embolus) blocking a distant
blood vessel

U71. bile pigment formed in liver from hemoglobin

V71. abnormal fluid-filled sac

W71. within normal limits

X71. muscle shortening due to spasm or fibrosis **

Y71. intestine-r

Z71. re muscle - attachment of muscle to a more movable part
of skeleton, as distinct from the origin

A72. detailed skin assessment tool

B72. pert to duodenum - 1st part of small intestine; 9-12 in
long

C72. creation -r

D72. pert to -s

E72. use of remedial proc to overcome a phys defect**
physiotherapy - another term for it

F72. inflamm of larynx, trachea, and bronchi

G72. turning eye away from its normal position *

H72. pert to tears and tear apparatus

I72. tailbone, at lowest end of vert column

J72. raised, irregular, lumpy scar due to excess collagen fiber
production during healing of a wound; (greek) stain

K72. wire mesh tube used to keep arteries open

L72. areas of pancreatic cells that prod insulin and glycagon

M72. region of pharynx (windpipe) at back of nose and above
soft palate *

N72. hormone prod by adrenal cortex

O72. larger bone of lower leg; latin - large shinbone

P72. excretion of large amounts of dilute urine as result of
inadequate antidiuretic hormone prod

Q72. r- solid

R72. r/cf - glue

S72. severe, malignant infect disease

T72. safety reminder device; eg. soft restraint

U72. purulent discharge

V72. pert to spaces between cells in a tissue or organ

W72. large red blood cell

X72. narrowing of a tube *

Y72. rapid breathing

Z72. the part of the trunk between the abdomen and neck

A73. terminal part of respiratory tract where gas exchange
occurs

B73. to lay flat or be overcome by physical weakness and
exhaustion; (latin) to stretch out

C73. endocrine gland in floor and wall of 3rd ventricle of
brain; prod 8 hormones

D73. to block, keep back -r

E73. compound liberated in tissues as result of injury or
immune response

F73. differential white blood count

G73. inflammatory skin disease, often with a serous discharge; (Greek) to boil or ferment

H73. break down food -r

I73. coal

J73. systematic tx of disease, dysfunc, or disorder **

K73. deficiency of ALL types of blood cells **

L73. muscle

M73. fleshy projection of the soft palate

N73. r-green

O73. condition -s

P73. uncontrolled quivering or twitching of the heart muscle

Q73. anus -r

R73. r-tooth

S73. cut, slice, layer

T73. r- to take up

U73. nonliving epidermis at base of fingernails

V73. paralysis of Both legs

W73. 1 of 2 div of autonomic nerv sys, calms the body, slows down heartbeat, stimulates digestion

X73. r- bladder

Y73. reg of pharynx at back of nose and aboe soft palate

Z73. away from - p

A74. having 2 points; bicuspid heart valve has 2 flaps **

B74. med spec of disorders of nervous system

C74. inside -p

D74. quality of -s

E74. flexion of a limb or part beyond normal limits

F74. colored portion of eye w/pupil in center

G74. abdominal region below the stomach

H74. organ system that covers the body; skin is the main orgain w/i the system;

I74. homrone that mobilizes glucose from body storage

J74. from -p

K74. endocrine gland located in mediastinum

L74. r- milk

M74. triangle-r

N74. hardening of the arteries

O74. mass of lymph tiss on either side of throat

P74. moving Toward a center

Q74. inherited disease from defic of clotting factor

R74. another name for pubic bone

S74. turn out -r

T74. seizures of children 5-10; stares vacantly for few seconds

U74. under, below, -p

V74. r - spine

W74. gluteus medius muscle is partly covered by gluteus maximus

X74. opening

Y74. r- nucleus

Z74. irritable bowel syndrome

A75. carbon dioxide

B75. humerus and radius

C75. r - diaphragm

D75. antibody- protein prod in response to an antigen

E75. resemble -s

F75. straight -r

G75. removing tissue from a living person for lab examination

H75. r- growth

I75. sebum -r

J75. resulting state -s

K75. pert to both the atrium and ventricle

L75. chemical formed in uncontrolled diabetes or in starvation

M75. llyph vessel carries chyle away from intestine

N75. total failure of healing of a fx

O75. lower and posterior part of hip bone

P75. nerve -r

Q75. mouth

R75. harmful, bad -r

Nursing Medical Terminology

Quiz

Med Terminol Quiz

Circle the letter of the Answer that corresponds to the displayed .

1. polyuria

    A. removal by suction of fluid or gas from a body cavity

    B. endocrine gland in floor an dwall of 3rd ventricle of brain; secretes feel-good hormone serotonin by day and converts it to melatonin at night

    C. r/cf - electricity

    D. excessive production of urine

2. perforation

    A. to block,

    B. blood vessel with oxygenated blood; carries blood away from heart

    C. dramatic form of seizue with: loc, eyes roll up, jaw clenched, may stop breathing

    D. hole thu wall of a structure

3. melan

    A. excessive, excess, above, beyond -p

    B. r- intestine

    C. black pigment -r

    D. most-s

4. tax

    A. point-r

    B. process-s

    C. r- coordination

    D. parasitic insect

5. tongue

    A. breakdown of complex substances into simpler ones as a part of metabolism

    B. mobile muscle mass in the mouth; has the taste buds *

    C. tumor, mass -s

    D. acute myocardial infarction - heart attack

6. voluntary muscle

    A. sensation of pain-r

    B. is under control of the will

    C. uncontrolled quivering or twitching of the heart muscle

    D. pertaining to the skin

7. mucocutaneous

    A. junction of skin and mucous membrane; (eg. the lips)

    B. fleshy projection of the soft palate

C. surgical excision -s

D. surg removal of adipose tissue using suction

8. pepsin

A. chamber of heart - pumps blood; also means a cavity in the brain (prod cerebrospinal fluid) **

B. enzyme prod by stomach that breaks down protein

C. collection of 7 bones in foot that form ankle and instep; latin - ankle

D. r- destroy

9. epistaxis

A. pubis -r

B. nose bleed

C. use of liquid nitrogen or argon gas in a probe to freeze and kill abnormal tissue

D. membrane that lines the interior of freely moving joints

10. endocrine

A. high BP

B. gland that pro internal or hormonal subst and secretes it into bllod;

C. inflammatory skin disease, often with a serous discharge; (Greek) to boil or ferment

D. chronic obstructive pulmonary disease; use Fowlers position

Circle the letter of the that corresponds to the displayed Answer.

11. analgesic and antipyetic (pain and fever)

A. acetaminophen

B. toxin

C. con

D. ing

12. tendon -r

A. tendin

B. zygoma

C. candida albicans

D. metabolism

13. terminal end of digestivve tract *

A. capsule

B. syn

C. anus

D. embolus

14. r - efficient, practical

A. melan

B. pract

C. abdomin

D. metatarsus

15. white blood cell
   A. maxilla
   B. WBC
   C. hyperpnea
   D. a

16. coronary vascular accident; stroke
   A. ing
   B. sigmoid
   C. ventricular arrhythmias include
   D. CVA

17. entrance, atrium -r
   A. insert
   B. bursa
   C. atri
   D. hemolysis

18. symptoms
   A. hypersplenism
   B. SX
   C. malabsorption
   D. occipit

19. r- chest
   A. hyperopia
   B. sphen
   C. thorax
   D. intussusception

20. touch, stroke-r
   A. palpat
   B. anterior
   C. ischemia
   D. murmur

EXTRA CREDIT: Give the that corresponds to the displayed Answer.

21. central portion of a structure surrounded by cortex, contains marrow; latin - marrow

Med Terminol Quiz

Circle the letter of the Answer that corresponds to the displayed .

1. respiratory

    A. bone is broken, but skin is not broken

    B. pertaining to respiration (breathing)

    C. inflammation of the skin and muscles

    D. study of structure and function of cells, tissues, and organs

2. tachycardia

    A. rapid heart rate, above 100 bpm

    B. r - change

    C. s- inflammation

    D. carries blood from intestines to liver

3. heart block

    A. occurs when interference in cardiac electrical conduction prevents atria's contraction from coordinating w/ventricles' contractions

    B. s - body

    C. together -p

    D. inflamm of tendon and its surrounding synovial sheath

4. abdominoplasty

    A. decreased blood volume in the body

    B. WBC w/multilobed nucleus

    C. tummy tuck; surgical removal of excess subcutaneous fat from abdominal wall

    D. body's prin carb reserve, stored in liver and skeletal muscle

5. nici

    A. fluid, noncellular part of blood

    B. lethal-r

    C. outer layer of the heart wall **

    D. blowing

6. sebum

    A. normal posterior curve of spine that can be exaggerated in disease

    B. touch, stroke-r

    C. waxy secretion of the sebaceous glands

    D. nosebleed

7. pulmonologist

    A. nose bleed

    B. skin-r

C. one -r

D. specialist studies the lungs

8. papill/o

A. papilla, pimple -r

B. endocrine gland in mediastinum

C. horizontal plane div body into uper and lower portions (superior and inferior)

D. r- solid

9. louse lice (pl)

A. diseasese

B. slipping of 1 part of bowel inside another to cause obstruction; telecoping **

C. cancer

D. parasitic insect

10. oma

A. r-enzyme, fermenting

B. tumor, mass -s

C. incise, cut -r

D. tarsal bone that articulates w/tibia to form the ankle joint; latin - heel bone

Circle the letter of the that corresponds to the displayed Answer.

11. surgical removal of adipose tissue

A. granulocyte

B. intracellular

C. lipectomy

D. AED

12. hard mass of cholseterol, calcium, and billirubin that can be formed in gb and bile duct

A. accomodation

B. al

C. gallstone

D. myop

13. backward -p

A. re

B. humoral immunity

C. fiber

D. fibroblast

14. nature-r

A. mammoplasty

B. tomy

C. phys

D. Tourette syndrome

15. skull
   A. cyst
   B. v-fib
   C. cranium
   D. accomodation

16. hemoglobin-red pigmented protein; main component of red blood cells
   A. caudal
   B. Hgb or Hb
   C. pod
   D. umbilical

17. mass of fibrin and cells that is prod in a wound
   A. clot
   B. tachypnea
   C. interventricular (IV)
   D. postnatal

18. intravenous
   A. IV
   B. acetaminophen
   C. exotropia
   D. coagulant

19. deeper and more rapid breathing than normal
   A. hernia
   B. hyperpnea
   C. CAD
   D. osteogenic sarcoma

20. myocardial infarct - heart attack
   A. brachi/i
   B. tomy
   C. sprain
   D. MI

EXTRA CREDIT: Give the that corresponds to the displayed Answer.

21. r- within

Med Terminol Quiz

Circle the letter of the Answer that corresponds to the displayed .

1. islets of Langerhans

    A. with, together-p

    B. areas of pancreatic cells that prod insulin and glycagon

    C. dissolve-s **

    D. fibrous band that connects muscle to bone; latin - sinew

2. thorax

    A. r- nearest to the center

    B. pert to tears and tear apparatus

    C. after

    D. r- chest

3. emuls

    A. take care of -r

    B. r- suspend in a liquid

    C. artificail opening into a tubular structure

    D. tendon -r

4. choledocholithisis

    A. * sudden, involuntary, repeated contraction of muscles

    B. r- pressure

    C. presence of gallstone in common bile duct

    D. wheezing sound heard on auscultation of lungs; made by air passing thru constricted lumen

5. nat

    A. make incapable of movement

    B. r- birth, born

    C. inability to focus light rays that enter the eye in different planes

    D. r- to lead

6. ile

    A. s- pertaining to

    B. r-ileum

    C. crescent, meniscus -r

    D. ringworm infections of the body's skin and hands

7. angiogram

    A. take care of -r

    B. to chew *

    C. radiograph obtained after injection of radiopaque contrast material into blood vess

    D. cell

8. scopy

    A. relating to stomach and duodenum

    B. process of using an instrument to examine visually

    C. sudden onset

    D. s- pertaining to

9. saliv

    A. r- saliva

    B. mouth of windpipe-r

    C. after

    D. raised, irregular, lumpy scar due to excess collagen fiber production during healing of a wound; (greek) stain

10. con

    A. detached piece of thrombus, a mass of bacteria, quantity of air, or foreign body that blocks a blood vessel

    B. with, together - p

    C. small terminal artery leading into capillary network

    D. s - pertaining to

Circle the letter of the that corresponds to the displayed Answer.

11. surg removal of a lung

    A. melanin

    B. pericarditis

    C. arrhythmia

    D. pneumonectomy

12. hormone secreted in stomach tath stim secretion of HCl and increases gastric motility

    A. gastrin

    B. cyanosis

    C. nucleus

    D. ceps

13. dx and tx of diseases of eye

    A. opthamology

    B. DVT

    C. CVA

    D. cardiomyopathy

14. substance capable of triggering an immune response

    A. membran

    B. antigen

    C. polyphagia

    D. ia

15. nose bleed

A. prognosis

B. pylor

C. regurgitate

D. epistaxis

16. r- accumulation of fluid

A. celi

B. rhonchus

C. congest

D. dorsi

17. smallest unit of the body capable of independent existence; (latin) storeroom

A. varices (sing-varix)

B. cell

C. pepsin

D. subcutaneus

18. oxygen -r

A. impetigo

B. intus

C. oxy

D. carbuncle

19. r- frenzy

A. man

B. parasite

C. dorsi

D. tox

20. acquired w/i a hospital

A. hypothalamus

B. nosocomial

C. glycer

D. scler/o

EXTRA CREDIT: Give the that corresponds to the displayed Answer.

21. strand or filament; latin -fiber

Med Terminol Quiz

Circle the letter of the Answer that corresponds to the displayed .

1. dors

    A. junction of skin and mucous membrane; (eg. the lips)

    B. patella -r

    C. s- pertaining to

    D. r - back

2. nervous tissue

    A. function: transmit impulses for coordination, sensory reception, motor actions; location- brain, spinal cord, nerves

    B. outer layer of the heart wall **

    C. sebum -r

    D. blood vessel

3. cartilage

    A. bone forms part of medial wall of orbit (around eye),

    B. volume-r

    C. nonvascular, firm connective tissue found mostly in joints; latin - gristle

    D. deficient levels of parathyroid hormone;

4. arthroscopy

    A. in front of the patella

    B. visual exam of interior of a joint

    C. 2 bones forming the side walls and roof of the cranium

    D. r- condition of intestine

5. macrocyte

    A. result of - s

    B. r-tongue

    C. chest -r

    D. large red blood cell

6. locat

    A. r-flow

    B. place -r

    C. skin eruption

    D. process of using an instrument to examine visually

7. thromb

    A. clot-r

    B. situated nearest the center of the body;situated closest to the point of attachment to the body, refers to limbs

C. tuberculosis

D. blood in pleural cavity

8. pronat

A. bend down-r

B. chest x-ray

C. decreased no of red blood cells

D. cell

9. colloid

A. forecast of the probable future course and outcome of a disease

B. liquid containing suspended particles

C. gland that secretes substances outwardly thru excretory ducts

D. violet, bluish-purple -r

10. py

A. black pigment -r

B. built up or put together from simpler compounds

C. r-pus

D. r- kidney

Circle the letter of the that corresponds to the displayed Answer.

11. p- half, derivied from hemi

A. incomplete freacture

B. percutaneous

C. mi

D. exocrine

12. fibrous band that connects muscle to bone

A. tendon

B. blast

C. insert

D. CXR

13. endocrine gland in floor and wall of 3rd ventricle of brain; prod 8 hormones

A. muscle

B. lacer

C. crine

D. hypothalamus

14. dark blue -r

A. laceration

B. periosteum

C. cyan (r)

D. heme

15. r- to lead
   A. anorexia
   B. duct
   C. excoriate
   D. osteopathy

16. muscle
   A. PDA
   B. phalanx, phalanges (pl)
   C. my
   D. rhin

17. without-par
   A. AMI
   B. epithelial tissue
   C. an
   D. etiology

18. coal
   A. anthrac (r)
   B. Kaposi sarcoma
   C. cruciate
   D. dislocation

19. complains of
   A. C/O
   B. hyperpyrexia
   C. pulmonary
   D. CA

20. tumor, mass-s
   A. cervic
   B. postnatal
   C. hyperpnea
   D. oma

EXTRA CREDIT: Give the that corresponds to the displayed Answer.

21. re muscle - attachment of muscle to a more movable part of skeleton, as distinct from the origin

Med Terminol Quiz

Circle the letter of the Answer that corresponds to the displayed .

1. virulence

    A. strength of pathogen

    B. r- shake or jar

    C. r- skull

    D. 2 bones joined by fibrocartilage; 2 pubic bones; greek - grow together

2. sebum

    A. wheezing sound heard on auscultation of lungs; made by air passing thru constricted lumen

    B. waxy secretion of the sebaceous glands

    C. a tissue consisting of cells that can contract

    D. major protein of connective tissue, cartilage, and bone

3. mucus

    A. finger or toe bones; 14 phalanges of hand- each finger has 3 joints except thumb which has only 2

    B. sticky secretion of cells in mucous membranes (Greek) slime

    C. take away-p

    D. detached piece of thrombus, mass of bacteria,air, or foreign body that blocks a blood vessel

4. PDA

    A. patent ductus arteriosus- an open, direct channel between aorta and pulmonary artery in newborn

    B. clear fluid collected from body tissues and transported by lymph vessells to the venous circulation; r-lymph,lymphatic system

    C. bone forms part of medial wall of orbit (around eye),

    D. pert to digestive tract

5. anter

    A. finger or toe bones; 14 phalanges of hand- each finger has 3 joints except thumb which has only 2

    B. other-p

    C. r - before

    D. systemic disease affecting many joints

6. sagittal

    A. artery-r

    B. vertical plane through the body divides it into right and left planes

    C. enlargement of the heart

    D. occurs when interference in cardiac electrical conduction prevents atria's contraction from coordinating w/ventricles' contractions

7. post

    A. triggered by fever in infants and toddlers 6 mos - 5 yrs, few dev epilepsy

    B. areas of pancreatic cells that prod insulin and glycagon

C. r- gums

D. p- after

8. hetero

A. rapid breathing

B. make incapable of movement

C. different -p

D. r-bitter

9. epidermis

A. tube that connects kidney to urinary bladder, (Greek) urinary canal, passage of urine

B. pert to nearer the tailbone; (same as inferior, opposite of cephalic)

C. top layer of skin

D. 1 of 4 regions of the surface of the abdomen; 1/4 of a circle,(latin) one quarter

10. cav

A. r- chest

B. pit in the abdomen where the umbilical cord entered the fetus

C. r - hollow space

D. passage thru skin, as by needle puncture

Circle the letter of the that corresponds to the displayed Answer.

11. congenital lesion of the skin; (latin) mole, birthmark

A. myringotomy

B. mucous

C. supine

D. nevus nevi (pl)

12. r- tear

A. A+O

B. papilla

C. macrocytic

D. lacrim

13. r- fully developed

A. bipolar disorder

B. mature

C. ly

D. number of bones in body

14. defense mech from antibodies in blood

A. lobe

B. humoral immunity

C. BS

D. gastr

15. artificial opening into a tubular structure; end of bowel opens into skin at a stoma; illeostomy, colostomy

   A. tendin
   B. ostomy
   C. linear fx
   D. petechia

16. r- beyond

   A. hyper
   B. dermatomyositis
   C. system
   D. otolith

17. the constantly changing physical and chemical rocesses occurring in the cell that are the sum of anabolism and catabolism

   A. pre
   B. metabolism
   C. physis
   D. or (os)

18. put together -r

   A. insert
   B. jejun
   C. scler
   D. centesis (r)

19. ability to see objects as they come into the outer edges of visual field

   A. vita
   B. glutin
   C. anastomosis
   D. peripheral vision

20. cancer -r

   A. micro
   B. IM
   C. carcin
   D. femor

EXTRA CREDIT: Give the that corresponds to the displayed Answer.

21. exam of contents of abdomen using endoscope

Nursing Medical Terminology

Test

Med Terminol Test

Enter the letter for the matching Answer

1. ☐ thorac
2. ☐ stasis
3. ☐ opsy
4. ☐ or
5. ☐ hyperflexion
6. ☐ WNL
7. ☐ excoriate
8. ☐ graine
9. ☐ calcaneus
10. ☐ scler/o
11. ☐ SX
12. ☐ tenosynovitis
13. ☐ -a
14. ☐ vertebra, vertebrae (pl)
15. ☐ de
16. ☐ protaglandin
17. ☐ pepsin
18. ☐ thromb
19. ☐ laryngotracheobronchitis
20. ☐ coron

A. r - chest

B. r-mouth

C. from, out of-p

D. r- head pain

E. hard

F. hormone present in many tissues, but first isolated from prostate gland

G. bone of tarsus (foot) that forms the heel

H. within normal limits

I. control, stop-s

J. inflamm of larynx, trachea, and bronchi

K. to view -s

L. blood clot-r

M. flexion of a limb or part beyond normal limits

N. r - crown

O. before

P. inflamm of tendon and its surrounding synovial sheath

Q. symptoms

R. to scratch

S. enzyme prod by stomach that breaks down protein

T. one of bones of spinal column

Give the Answer that corresponds to the displayed .

21. amin

22. embol

23. AC

Give the that corresponds to the displayed Answer.

24.   the process of building a compound from different elements

25.   bone -r

26.   nose bleed

27.   r- nearest to the center

28.   inflammation of lung parenchyma tissue

29.   part of capsule of the shoulder joint **

30.   reconstitution, rebuilding of a lost part

Med Terminol Test

Enter the letter for the matching Answer

1. ☐ bari
2. ☐ linear fx
3. ☐ nucle/o
4. ☐ macrocyte
5. ☐ CDiff
6. ☐ sebaceous glands
7. ☐ meniscus
8. ☐ rrhea
9. ☐ kyphosis
10. ☐ atelectasis
11. ☐ endo
12. ☐ physis
13. ☐ myel
14. ☐ congest
15. ☐ cortic
16. ☐ quadrant
17. ☐ bilirubin
18. ☐ Alzheihmer disease
19. ☐ a
20. ☐ mucus

A. humpbacked condition

B. form of dementia; nvervecells inareas of brain assoc w/memory and cognition are replaced by abnormal protein clumps and tangles

C. fx runs parallel to the long axis of the bone

D. weight -r

E. r-flow

F. r- spinal cord

G. disc of cartilage between the bones of the joint (eg. at knee cap); (latin) cresent

H. r/cf - nucleus

I. Clostridium Difficile - very contageous diahhrea; contact isolation - gown,gloves

J. r- growth

K. large red blood cell

L. 1 of 4 regions of the surface of the abdomen; 1/4 of a circle,(latin) one quarter

M. cortex -r

N. located in the dermis that open into hair follicles and secrete a waxy fluid called sebum

O. collapse of part of lung

P. within - p

Q. without -p

R. bile pigment formed in liver from hemoglobin

S. r- accumulation of fluid

T. sticky secretion o f cells in mucous membranes

Give the Answer that corresponds to the displayed .

21. ate

22. UTI

23. prn

24. crete

Give the that corresponds to the displayed Answer.

25. nonvascular, firm connective tissue found mostly in joints; (latin) gristle

26. self gov visceral motor div of peripheral nerv sys

27. occurs when interference in cardiac electrical conduction prevents atria's contraction from coordinating w/ventricles' contractions

28. backward flow; (latin)backward flow

29. cond having gallstones (bile stones) *

30. surgicqally made union between 2 tubular structures

Med Terminol Test

Enter the letter for the matching Answer

1. ☐ blast
2. ☐ pronation
3. ☐ posterior
4. ☐ leukocytosis
5. ☐ hypertrophy
6. ☐ HCl
7. ☐ pelv
8. ☐ paraplegia
9. ☐ pediculosis
10. ☐ IDDM
11. ☐ clavicul
12. ☐ tarsus
13. ☐ palate
14. ☐ nosocomial
15. ☐ interventricular (IV)
16. ☐ therap
17. ☐ hiatus
18. ☐ emphysema
19. ☐ uterus
20. ☐ microcyte

A. dilation of respiratory bronchiles and alveoli

B. small red blood cell

C. increase in size, but not in number, of an indiv tissue element **

D. pertaining to the back surface of the body, situated behind

E. collection of 7 bones in foot that form ankle and instep; latin - ankle

F. roof of mouth, floor of nose

G. organ in which an egg develops into fetus; (latin) womb

H. opening thru a structure

I. insuline dependent diabetes mellitus; type 1 diabetes,

J. clavicle -r

K. paralysis of Both legs

L. acid of gastric juice

M. r - pelvis

N. immature cell-s

O. between ventricles of the heart

P. excessive number of WBCs

Q. acquired w/i a hospital

R. r- treatment

S. an infection with lice

T. proc of lying face down on belly position, or turning a hand or foot with volar (palm or sole) surface down

Give the Answer that corresponds to the displayed .

21. WNL

22. ceps

23. cyst

Give the that corresponds to the displayed Answer.

24. sore caused by lying down for long periods of time

25. state of muscular contraction *

26. cavity or hollow space in bone or other tissue

27. athlete's foot

28. insertion of needle into pleural cavity to withdraw fluid or air

29. compound liberated in tissues as result of injury or immune response

30. patholic compression of an organ, such as the heart

Med Terminol Test

1. ☐ ICD
2. ☐ lyt
3. ☐ meninges
4. ☐ ileostomy
5. ☐ oral
6. ☐ emuls
7. ☐ axilla
8. ☐ heart block
9. ☐ keratin
10. ☐ skelet
11. ☐ py
12. ☐ IV
13. ☐ triglyceride
14. ☐ de
15. ☐ LDL
16. ☐ NSAID
17. ☐ um
18. ☐ toxin
19. ☐ MRSA
20. ☐ anabolism

A. buildup of complex substances in the cell from simpler ones as a part of metabolism

B. 3 layered covering of the brain and spinal cord *

C. occurs when interference in cardiac electrical conduction prevents atria's contraction from coordinating w/ventricles' contractions

D. r-pus

E. artificial opening from ileum to outside of body

F. protein present in skin, hair, and nails

G. implantable cardioverter/defibrillator- sense abnormal rhythms; gives heart small shock to return rhythm to normal

H. from, out of-p

I. Methicillin Resistant Stapholococus Aureus- extremely virulent staph infection, can be fatal; use contact isolation - gloves and gown

J. armpit

K. low density lipoprotein- bad cholesterol

L. poinsonous substance formed by a cell or organism;

M. skeleton -r

N. pert to mouth

O. lipid containing 3 fatty acids

P. nonsteroidal anti-inflammatory drug

Q. structure

R. destroy-r

S. r- suspend in a liquid

T. intravenous

Give the Answer that corresponds to the displayed .

21. glyc

22. syn

23. de

24. the process of building a compound from different elements

25. inability to focus light rays that enter the eye in different planes

26. immune rxn directed against person's own tissue

27. an infection with lice

28. pert to spaces between cells in a tissue or organ

29. presence of persecutory delusions

30. r- eardrum

Med Terminol Test

Enter the letter for the matching Answer

1. ☐ lyze
2. ☐ ation
3. ☐ intra
4. ☐ blast
5. ☐ retrovirus
6. ☐ gen
7. ☐ kerat
8. ☐ cellulitis
9. ☐ arthr/o
10. ☐ radius
11. ☐ cholelithiasis
12. ☐ in
13. ☐ globin
14. ☐ laser surgery
15. ☐ visual acuity
16. ☐ pectoral
17. ☐ ize
18. ☐ mania
19. ☐ articulate
20. ☐ enzyme

A. immature cell

B. creation -r

C. process -s

D. virus w/RNA core

E. use of concentrated, intense narrow beam of electromagnetic radiation for surg

F. mood disorder w/hperactivity, irritability, and rapid speech

G. cond having gallstones (bile stones) *

H. protein that induces changes in other substances

I. hard protein -r

J. protein-r

K. affect in a specific way -s

L. p- within

M. 2 separate bones have formed a joint

N. joint -r

O. inflammation of subcutaneous connective tissue

P. pert to chest **

Q. forearm bone on the thumb side; latin - spoke of a wheel

R. substance -s

S. r- destroy

T. * sharpness and clearness of vision

Give the Answer that corresponds to the displayed .

21. WNV

22. ventr

23. sten/o

24. trophy

25. SX

26. SQ

Give the that corresponds to the displayed Answer.

27. tube linking pharynx and stomach

28. * inflammation of meninges, bacterial or viral; vaccination available !

29. causes warts and is associated with cancer

30. pertaining to the cevix, or to the neck region